Living in Balance

Living in Balance

Matthew Petchinsky

Living in Balance: A Comprehensive Survival Guide to Thriving with Diabetes Insipidus

By: Matthew Petchinsky

Introduction

Overview of Diabetes Insipidus (DI)

Diabetes Insipidus (DI) is a rare but impactful condition characterized by the body's inability to regulate water balance effectively. Unlike diabetes mellitus, which involves high blood sugar levels due to issues with insulin production or use, DI is defined by excessive thirst (polydipsia) and the excretion of large amounts of diluted urine (polyuria). This imbalance is due to the kidneys' inability to conserve water, a function usually governed by antidiuretic hormone (ADH), also known as vasopressin.

DI is categorized into four main types, each with unique causes and characteristics:

- **Central Diabetes Insipidus (CDI)**: The most common form, CDI results from a deficiency of ADH production or release due to damage to the hypothalamus or pituitary gland. Such damage can be caused by head injuries, tumors, infections, or genetic disorders.

- **Nephrogenic Diabetes Insipidus (NDI)**: In NDI, the kidneys are unable to respond to ADH properly, even though it is produced at normal levels. This condition can be inherited or acquired through chronic kidney disease, certain medications (such as lithium), or metabolic imbalances.

- **Gestational Diabetes Insipidus**: This temporary form occurs during pregnancy when the placenta produces an enzyme that breaks down ADH. It typically resolves after childbirth but requires monitoring to prevent complications during pregnancy.

- **Dipsogenic Diabetes Insipidus**: This less common type is caused by a defect in the thirst mechanism, leading to excessive water intake that suppresses ADH production. It can be triggered by certain mental health conditions, trauma, or structural abnormalities in the hypothalamus.

Understanding these types is crucial for recognizing how DI affects individuals differently and why specific treatment plans are necessary for effective management.

Understanding Water Balance

Water is essential for the body's physiological functions, including maintaining body temperature, joint lubrication, waste elimination, and cellular health. The kidneys play a central role in regulating water balance, primarily through the action of ADH.

ADH is produced by the hypothalamus and stored and released by the pituitary gland. Its function is to signal the kidneys to reabsorb water back into the bloodstream rather than excreting it as urine. When ADH binds to receptors in the kidneys, it increases the permeability of the collecting ducts, allowing more water to be reabsorbed and thereby concentrating the urine.

In a healthy individual, this mechanism ensures that water loss and intake remain balanced. However, in individuals with DI, this regulatory process is impaired:

- **Central DI**: Insufficient production or release of ADH means that even if the body needs to conserve water, the kidneys do not receive the signal to do so.
- **Nephrogenic DI**: The kidneys do not respond appropriately to ADH, regardless of its presence, leading to excessive water loss.
- **Gestational DI**: During pregnancy, an enzyme from the placenta can degrade ADH, disrupting water balance temporarily.
- **Dipsogenic DI**: Abnormal thirst leads to excessive water intake, which dilutes blood sodium levels and suppresses natural ADH production, disrupting kidney function.

When these processes are disrupted, the body experiences frequent urination and unrelenting thirst, leading to potential dehydration and electrolyte imbalances. Understanding this mechanism lays the groundwork for managing DI effectively.

Purpose of the Guide

Navigating life with Diabetes Insipidus can be challenging, but with the right information and strategies, it is possible to maintain a high quality of life. This guide, **"Living in Balance: A Comprehensive Survival Guide to Thriving with Diabetes Insipidus,"** aims to be a trusted companion for anyone affected by this condition—whether you are newly diagnosed, a long-time DI patient, or a caregiver.

What This Guide Offers:

- **Practical Advice and Management Strategies**: From hydration techniques and dietary advice to emergency preparedness and mental health support, this guide covers all aspects of living with DI.
- **Comprehensive Insights**: Clear explanations of the underlying mechanisms of DI, treatment options, and differences between each type help readers understand their condition better.
- **Supportive Resources**: Recommendations for financial management, insurance navigation, support networks, and advocacy provide an extra layer of practical assistance.
- **Child and Family-Focused Information**: Special considerations for managing DI in children and helping families adjust to the lifestyle changes necessary for effective care.
- **Tools for Empowerment**: Sample logs, checklists, and real-life advice empower readers to take control of their health and daily routines.

Living with DI requires adaptation, resilience, and informed decisions. This guide's purpose is to make that journey easier by equipping you with the knowledge and tools needed to handle every aspect of the condition confidently and effectively. Whether you need insights on medications, strategies for travel, or tips for balancing daily hydration, this guide is designed to help you thrive while maintaining balance in your life.

Chapter 1: Identifying the Signs – Recognizing Symptoms Early

Recognizing the early signs of Diabetes Insipidus (DI) is essential for timely diagnosis and effective management. Understanding these indicators not only facilitates early medical intervention but also reduces the risk of complications such as severe dehydration and electrolyte imbalance. In this chapter, we'll delve deeply into the primary symptoms of DI and explore how they present in individuals across different types of DI.

1.1 Excessive Thirst (Polydipsia)

One of the hallmark symptoms of DI is an unrelenting and insatiable thirst, known as polydipsia. This type of thirst is different from the kind experienced after physical activity or hot weather—it is persistent and often requires an unusually large amount of water intake to feel temporarily quenched.

- **What Triggers Polydipsia?** In DI, the body's inability to retain water triggers continuous signals to the brain, prompting excessive thirst as a compensatory response.
- **Characteristics of Thirst in DI**: Individuals with DI may consume several liters of water daily (often up to 10-15 liters), far exceeding the normal water intake of about 2-3 liters per day for healthy adults.
- **Impact on Daily Life**: This excessive thirst can disrupt daily activities, leading individuals to constantly seek out water, which may interfere with work, school, and social interactions.

1.2 Frequent Urination (Polyuria)

Accompanying the intense thirst is polyuria, or the production of abnormally large amounts of diluted urine. This symptom is often the most noticeable and can be distressing due to its frequency and volume.

- **Volume and Frequency**: Patients with DI may produce up to 15-20 liters of urine per day. This significantly exceeds the average adult's normal urine output of approximately 1-2 liters daily.
- **Characteristics of Urine**: The urine in DI is typically very diluted, appearing almost colorless due to the high water content and low concentration of solutes.
- **Nighttime Urination (Nocturia)**: Polyuria often extends into the night, leading to frequent awakenings to urinate (nocturia). This symptom disrupts sleep and can contribute to fatigue and reduced overall well-being.
- **Quality of Life Impact**: Frequent urination can interfere with an individual's ability to participate in daily activities, travel, or even sleep through the night uninterrupted. These disruptions can have downstream effects on mental health and daily functioning.

1.3 Dehydration Risks

Despite the body's compensatory mechanisms of excessive drinking and urination, dehydration remains a significant risk for those with untreated or poorly managed DI.

- **Mechanisms of Dehydration**: When the body loses water faster than it can be replenished, dehydration sets in. This is particularly concerning in DI because the kidneys do not conserve water effectively, even when the body needs to retain fluids.
- **Signs of Dehydration**: Symptoms of dehydration include:

  ○ Dry mouth and mucous membranes
  ○ Reduced skin elasticity
  ○ Sunken eyes
  ○ Fatigue and lethargy
  ○ Dizziness or lightheadedness
  ○ Rapid heart rate

- **Complications from Dehydration**: Severe dehydration can lead to an imbalance of electrolytes, which are critical for proper muscle function and nerve communication. This imbalance may cause muscle cramps, confusion, and, in extreme cases, seizures or unconsciousness.
- **High-Risk Situations**: Certain conditions can exacerbate the risk of dehydration, including hot weather, physical exertion, or periods of limited water access.

1.4 Other Associated Symptoms

While excessive thirst and urination are the most prominent indicators of DI, there are additional symptoms and signs that may be present, depending on the type and severity of the condition:

- **Unexplained Weight Loss**: Due to the substantial water loss, individuals may experience noticeable weight loss that is unrelated to changes in diet or physical activity.
- **Dry Skin and Cracked Lips**: Persistent water loss leads to dryness of the skin and lips. These outward signs can be early clues that hydration is insufficient despite high water intake.
- **Headaches**: Chronic dehydration can contribute to frequent headaches, which may be confused with tension or other types of headaches if the underlying cause is not identified.
- **Irritability and Mood Changes**: Dehydration and poor sleep due to frequent nocturia can lead to irritability, anxiety, and mood disturbances.

- **Fatigue**: The body's constant need to process large volumes of water and the disrupted sleep cycle due to nocturia can cause chronic fatigue and reduced energy levels.

1.5 Recognizing Symptoms in Children

DI can present differently in children, who may not be able to articulate their symptoms clearly. Early detection in pediatric cases is crucial to prevent developmental delays and complications:

- **Key Indicators in Infants**:
  - Unusually wet diapers and frequent urination
  - Excessive crying due to thirst
  - Vomiting and failure to thrive
- **Indicators in Older Children**:
  - Bed-wetting (enuresis) beyond the usual age
  - Difficulty focusing in school due to fatigue or disrupted sleep
  - Persistent requests for water throughout the day

1.6 When to Seek Medical Attention

Recognizing when these symptoms warrant medical attention is vital for early intervention:

- **Red Flags**: Persistent thirst and urination that disrupt daily life, signs of dehydration despite high water intake, and unexplained weight loss should be evaluated by a healthcare professional.
- **Consultation and Diagnosis**: Seeking medical evaluation early can facilitate diagnosis through appropriate tests, such as urine concentration tests, blood analysis, and water deprivation tests, which help distinguish DI from other conditions with similar symptoms.

Understanding these key indicators and taking note of how they manifest is the first step toward effectively managing and treating Diabetes Insipidus. Early recognition can lead to prompt medical intervention, improving outcomes and quality of life for those affected by this rare condition.

Chapter 2: Getting Answers – Diagnosis and Working with Your Healthcare Team

Receiving an accurate diagnosis is the cornerstone for effective management of Diabetes Insipidus (DI). Early detection and a clear understanding of the condition ensure that individuals can take steps toward appropriate treatment and improved quality of life. This chapter outlines the diagnostic process, details key medical tests involved, and emphasizes the importance of assembling a supportive healthcare team.

2.1 Steps in Diagnosing Diabetes Insipidus

The diagnostic journey for DI involves a series of systematic steps. Due to the overlapping symptoms with other conditions, a thorough evaluation is necessary to differentiate DI from other disorders that cause excessive thirst and urination, such as diabetes mellitus and psychogenic polydipsia.

Step 1: Medical History and Symptom Discussion

- **Initial Consultation**: The diagnostic process typically begins with an in-depth conversation with a healthcare provider, where patients share their medical history, current symptoms, and any family history of similar issues.
- **Detailed Symptom Log**: Keeping a record of the frequency of urination, water intake, and associated symptoms such as fatigue or nocturia can provide valuable insights for the physician.

Step 2: Physical Examination

- **Basic Assessment**: A physical examination helps identify any signs of dehydration or other physical manifestations related to DI, such as dry skin or sunken eyes.
- **Evaluation of General Health**: The doctor may assess body weight, blood pressure, and heart rate to evaluate overall health and hydration status.

Step 3: Preliminary Laboratory Tests

- **Blood Tests**: Basic blood tests are ordered to measure levels of electrolytes such as sodium and potassium. Elevated sodium levels are common in DI due to water loss, while other blood components help differentiate between types of DI and rule out diabetes mellitus.
- **Urine Analysis**: A urine sample is analyzed to measure osmolality (the concentration of urine). In individuals with DI, the urine is usually very dilute, with a low osmolality despite high urine volume.

2.2 Key Diagnostic Tests for Confirming DI

Accurate diagnosis often requires more specialized tests to determine the type of DI and guide treatment.

Water Deprivation Test

- **Purpose**: The water deprivation test is a critical diagnostic tool for assessing how well the kidneys conserve water when fluid intake is restricted.
- **Procedure**: Under close medical supervision, the patient stops drinking fluids for several hours while urine output and blood osmolality are monitored. Weight, blood pressure, and vital signs are also checked periodically.
- **Interpretation**: In healthy individuals, urine becomes more concentrated during dehydration. However, in cases of DI, the urine remains dilute even as dehydration progresses, confirming the diagnosis.
- **ADH Administration**: In the latter part of the test, synthetic ADH (desmopressin) may be administered. If urine concentration improves after administration, it suggests central DI. If there is no change, nephrogenic DI is likely.

ADH Level Blood Test

- **Purpose**: Measuring the level of antidiuretic hormone in the blood can help determine whether the body is producing an adequate amount of ADH.
- **Interpretation**: Low ADH levels indicate central DI, whereas normal or high ADH levels, coupled with a poor response to the hormone, suggest nephrogenic DI.

Magnetic Resonance Imaging (MRI)

- **Purpose**: An MRI scan of the brain may be ordered to identify any abnormalities in the hypothalamus or pituitary gland, such as tumors or structural changes that could affect ADH production.
- **Procedure**: The non-invasive scan provides detailed images of brain tissues and helps pinpoint potential causes of central DI.

Genetic Testing

- **Purpose**: In cases where nephrogenic DI is suspected, especially in children or those with a family history, genetic testing can identify mutations in the genes that affect kidney response to ADH.
- **Procedure**: A simple blood sample or cheek swab is used to analyze DNA for specific genetic markers.

2.3 Differentiating Between Types of DI

Correctly identifying the type of DI is crucial, as it affects treatment approaches:

- **Central DI**: Confirmed when there is a significant response to desmopressin during the water deprivation test. MRI may reveal structural anomalies in the hypothalamus or pituitary gland.
- **Nephrogenic DI**: Indicated when there is no response to desmopressin. This type may require further testing to uncover underlying causes such as medication side effects or chronic kidney disease.
- **Gestational DI**: Usually diagnosed based on symptoms that occur during pregnancy and may require a more nuanced approach, including monitoring and blood tests to assess ADH levels.
- **Dipsogenic DI**: Determined by ruling out other forms and identifying abnormal thirst regulation through patient history and specialized tests.

2.4 Building a Comprehensive Healthcare Team

Effective management of DI extends beyond diagnosis; it requires a dedicated healthcare team for ongoing support. The right team can ensure continuous monitoring, treatment optimization, and support through lifestyle changes.

Primary Care Physician (PCP)

- **Role**: The PCP is often the first point of contact and plays a crucial role in coordinating care, conducting initial evaluations, and managing general health.

Endocrinologist

- **Role**: As specialists in hormone-related conditions, endocrinologists are essential for the diagnosis and treatment of DI. They interpret test results, prescribe medications, and provide long-term disease management plans.

Nephrologist

- **Role**: A nephrologist may be involved in cases of nephrogenic DI or when kidney function is affected. They help adjust treatment plans and manage complications related to kidney health.

Dietitian/Nutritionist

- **Role**: Proper nutrition and hydration strategies are vital for DI management. A dietitian can provide personalized dietary plans that include balanced electrolytes and fluids, supporting overall health and minimizing dehydration risks.

Mental Health Professional

- **Role**: The challenges of living with a chronic condition like DI can impact mental health. A psychologist or counselor can offer coping strategies for managing stress, anxiety, and sleep disruptions associated with frequent nocturia and daily symptom management.

Pharmacist

- **Role**: Pharmacists are key in providing guidance on medication use, potential side effects, and interactions with other drugs, helping ensure patients receive maximum benefit from prescribed treatments.

2.5 Building Your Support Network

Support does not end with healthcare professionals. Building a network that includes family, friends, and peer support groups can greatly enhance quality of life:

- **Family and Friends**: Educating loved ones about DI can foster understanding and provide practical help with managing symptoms and lifestyle adjustments.
- **Peer Support Groups**: Online and in-person groups offer a space to share experiences, learn from others, and receive emotional support.
- **Patient Advocacy Organizations**: Nonprofit groups can provide resources, information, and advocacy for DI patients, connecting them with additional services and support networks.

Diagnosing and managing DI requires thorough examination, collaborative care, and continuous support. By following the steps outlined and leveraging the expertise of a robust healthcare team, patients can achieve effective symptom management and lead fulfilling lives.

Chapter 3: Managing Medications – An Overview of DI Treatments

Effective management of Diabetes Insipidus (DI) often relies on a tailored treatment plan involving medication. This chapter provides an in-depth overview of the most common medications used in the treatment of DI, their mechanisms of action, and considerations for each type of DI. Understanding how these treatments work and their implications is crucial for optimal symptom management and quality of life.

3.1 Desmopressin (DDAVP) – The Gold Standard for Central DI

Desmopressin (DDAVP) is the most widely used medication for the treatment of Central Diabetes Insipidus (CDI). It is a synthetic analog of the natural antidiuretic hormone (ADH) vasopressin and works by increasing water reabsorption in the kidneys, thereby reducing urine output and alleviating excessive thirst.

How Desmopressin Works:

- **Mechanism of Action**: Desmopressin binds to the V2 receptors in the kidneys' collecting ducts, prompting water retention and resulting in more concentrated urine.
- **Forms of Administration**: Desmopressin is available in several forms, including oral tablets, nasal spray, and injectable solutions, allowing flexibility in how it is taken based on patient needs and preferences.
- **Dosage and Timing**: The dose and frequency depend on the severity of symptoms and individual response to the medication. Most patients take it once or twice a day, typically in the morning and before bedtime.

Considerations and Side Effects:

- **Hyponatremia Risk**: One of the most significant risks associated with desmopressin is hyponatremia (low blood sodium levels), which can occur if the body retains too much water. This can lead to symptoms such as headache, nausea, confusion, or even seizures in severe cases.
- **Monitoring**: Regular monitoring of blood sodium levels is essential, especially when starting or adjusting the dosage. Patients are advised to limit fluid intake when taking desmopressin to avoid water intoxication.
- **Adherence**: Consistency in medication use and adherence to prescribed doses are critical for maintaining the delicate balance between hydration and electrolyte levels.

3.2 Thiazide Diuretics – Counterintuitive but Effective for Nephrogenic DI

While diuretics are typically used to increase urine output, thiazide diuretics are paradoxically beneficial in treating Nephrogenic Diabetes Insipidus (NDI). Thiazides work by reducing the amount of urine produced and helping to maintain water balance.

How Thiazide Diuretics Work:

- **Mechanism of Action**: Thiazide diuretics decrease the amount of fluid filtered by the kidneys, reducing urine volume and promoting sodium reabsorption, which helps maintain water balance.
- **Common Types**: Hydrochlorothiazide is a frequently prescribed thiazide diuretic for NDI.

Considerations and Side Effects:

- **Electrolyte Imbalance**: Thiazides can cause imbalances in electrolytes, including potassium. Patients may need to monitor their levels regularly and adjust their diet or take supplements as needed.
- **Combination Therapy**: Thiazides are often used in combination with other medications, such as nonsteroidal anti-inflammatory drugs (NSAIDs), to enhance their effectiveness.
- **Hydration Management**: While thiazides help reduce urine output, it is still important for patients to monitor hydration levels carefully to avoid dehydration.

3.3 Nonsteroidal Anti-Inflammatory Drugs (NSAIDs) – Enhancing Diuretic Effects

NSAIDs, such as indomethacin, can be used as an adjunct treatment for Nephrogenic DI. These medications help reduce urine volume by decreasing kidney filtration and enhancing the effects of thiazide diuretics.

How NSAIDs Work:

- **Mechanism of Action**: NSAIDs inhibit prostaglandin production, which reduces renal blood flow and decreases the amount of urine produced.
- **Usage**: NSAIDs are typically prescribed as part of a combination treatment plan with thiazide diuretics.

Considerations and Side Effects:

- **Potential Side Effects**: Long-term use of NSAIDs can lead to gastrointestinal issues, kidney damage, and increased risk of cardiovascular problems. Therefore, they should be used under close supervision.

- **Monitoring**: Regular kidney function tests are essential for patients on NSAID therapy to prevent potential damage.

3.4 Amiloride – A Potassium-Sparing Diuretic for Specific Cases

Amiloride is a diuretic that is particularly useful in cases of NDI caused by lithium toxicity, as it helps counteract the effects of lithium on the kidneys.

How Amiloride Works:

- **Mechanism of Action**: Amiloride blocks sodium channels in the kidneys, reducing sodium reabsorption and promoting water retention, thus decreasing urine output.
- **Benefits for Lithium-Induced NDI**: This medication can help restore the kidney's response to ADH and improve overall water balance in patients with lithium-induced NDI.

Considerations and Side Effects:

- **Potassium Levels**: Amiloride is a potassium-sparing diuretic, meaning it does not cause potassium loss. However, patients should monitor their potassium levels to avoid hyperkalemia (excessively high potassium).
- **Side Effects**: Common side effects include gastrointestinal discomfort and dizziness. Patients should report any severe reactions to their healthcare provider.

3.5 Hormonal Treatments for Gestational DI

Gestational DI is a temporary condition that can develop during pregnancy due to the increased breakdown of ADH by an enzyme produced by the placenta. Treatment typically involves desmopressin, which is safe for both the mother and baby when monitored properly.

Special Considerations:

- **Dosage Adjustments**: Hormonal changes during pregnancy may require adjustments to the dosage of desmopressin.
- **Monitoring**: Regular monitoring of blood sodium levels is particularly important during pregnancy to ensure both maternal and fetal health.

3.6 Supportive Treatments and Lifestyle Considerations

While medications play a critical role in managing DI, lifestyle adjustments and supportive treatments can enhance their effectiveness and improve overall well-being.

Dietary Adjustments:

- **Low-Sodium Diet**: Reducing sodium intake can help decrease urine output, particularly in patients with NDI. A low-sodium diet can also support the effectiveness of thiazide diuretics.
- **Hydration Strategies**: Patients must strike a balance between staying hydrated and avoiding excessive fluid intake, which could lead to water intoxication when on desmopressin.

Monitoring and Logging:

- **Symptom and Intake Logs**: Keeping a detailed record of water intake, urine output, and any symptoms can help healthcare providers make informed decisions regarding treatment adjustments.

- **Routine Check-Ups**: Regular follow-ups with an endocrinologist or nephrologist are essential to monitor the effectiveness of treatment and make necessary adjustments.

Emergency Preparedness:

- **Emergency Kits**: Patients should have a readily accessible emergency kit with medications, contact information for their healthcare team, and instructions for emergency situations where they might become dehydrated or need urgent treatment.
- **Medical Alert Identification**: Wearing a medical alert bracelet or carrying an ID card that states the individual has DI can be lifesaving in emergency scenarios.

3.7 Personalized Treatment Plans

Treatment for DI is not one-size-fits-all. Each patient's plan should be tailored to their specific type of DI, the severity of their symptoms, and their overall health status.

Collaborative Approach:

- **Coordination with Specialists**: Effective management often requires collaboration among primary care physicians, endocrinologists, nephrologists, dietitians, and mental health professionals.
- **Patient Involvement**: Patients should be active participants in their care, understanding their medication plan, potential side effects, and when to seek help.

Regular Re-Evaluations:

- **Adjusting Treatment**: As life circumstances change, such as during pregnancy or with the onset of new medical conditions, treatment plans may need adjustment.
- **Advocating for Your Health**: Patients should feel empowered to discuss any concerns or changes in symptoms with their healthcare providers to ensure their treatment plan continues to meet their needs.

Effective medication management is fundamental for living with DI. By understanding the available treatment options, their mechanisms, and considerations for use, patients can work closely with their healthcare team to find the most suitable and sustainable plan for their condition.

Chapter 4: Staying Hydrated – Essential Water Intake Strategies

Maintaining proper hydration is a cornerstone of managing Diabetes Insipidus (DI). Unlike typical hydration practices, individuals with DI need tailored strategies that address their unique challenges: balancing the high volume of urine output with adequate fluid intake while avoiding potential risks like dehydration and hyponatremia. In this chapter, we explore practical and detailed tips for managing hydration effectively, ensuring safe water intake, and controlling unrelenting thirst.

4.1 Understanding Hydration Needs in DI

People with DI can lose up to 15-20 liters of urine per day, much higher than the 1-2 liters typical in healthy adults. This massive fluid loss makes proper hydration essential to prevent dehydration and electrolyte imbalances.

Key Points:

- **Fluid Intake vs. Fluid Loss**: The primary goal is to match fluid intake with urine output to maintain an equilibrium in the body.
- **Signs of Dehydration**: Knowing the early signs—such as dry mouth, headaches, dizziness, and decreased skin elasticity—helps in quick intervention.

4.2 Strategies for Maintaining Hydration

Proper hydration requires consistency and mindful practices. The following strategies are designed to help individuals with DI stay hydrated without risking overhydration:

1. Structured Hydration Schedule

- **Pre-set Intervals**: Establish regular times throughout the day to drink water rather than waiting for thirst to build up excessively. This helps maintain steady hydration levels.

- **Morning Hydration Boost**: Start the day with a significant amount of water to replenish fluids lost overnight, but avoid drinking too much at once to prevent overloading the kidneys.
- **Nighttime Management**: For individuals affected by nocturia (frequent urination at night), balancing hydration in the evening is critical. Reduce fluid intake a few hours before bedtime but ensure sufficient hydration earlier in the evening.

2. Small, Frequent Sips vs. Large Amounts

- **Frequent Sipping**: Drinking small sips throughout the day is more effective than consuming large volumes at once, as it helps the body absorb water gradually without overwhelming the kidneys.
- **Avoid Chugging Water**: Rapidly drinking large amounts can increase the risk of water intoxication, particularly when taking medications like desmopressin.

3. Electrolyte Balance

- **Hydration Isn't Just Water**: Incorporating electrolyte solutions can help maintain a balance between water intake and essential minerals like sodium and potassium.
- **Use Oral Rehydration Solutions (ORS)**: These solutions contain a balanced mix of water, salts, and sugar to facilitate absorption and prevent electrolyte depletion.
- **Homemade Solutions**: Mix a pinch of salt, a small amount of sugar, and water to create a simple, effective rehydration drink.

4.3 Safe Water Intake Practices

Safety in hydration goes beyond simply drinking enough water. Patients with DI need to manage how and when they consume fluids to avoid complications like hyponatremia.

1. Monitor Water Intake and Output

- **Use a Hydration Log**: Keeping a detailed log of daily water intake and urine output can help you and your healthcare provider adjust your hydration strategy.
- **Digital Tools**: Consider using hydration tracking apps or devices that can log fluid intake and alert you to drink water at set intervals.

2. Limit Fluid Intake with Desmopressin Use

- **Fluid Restriction**: When taking desmopressin, excessive water intake can lead to water retention and hyponatremia (low sodium levels). Limiting fluid intake to match what your body needs helps prevent complications.
- **Guidelines from Your Doctor**: Work closely with your doctor to establish safe limits on fluid consumption based on your medication dose and daily activity level.

3. Recognize Thirst Cues

- **Understanding True vs. Habitual Thirst**: People with DI often develop a habit of constantly drinking due to their condition. Learning to differentiate between true thirst and habitual drinking can help prevent overhydration.

- **Mindful Drinking**: Drink water mindfully, focusing on whether you truly feel thirsty or are drinking out of routine.

4. Stay Cool in Hot Weather

- **Cooling Techniques**: In hot or humid conditions, body temperature regulation becomes more critical. Use cooling towels, fans, and air conditioning to minimize the need for excessive water consumption.
- **Cold Water and Ice Chips**: Sipping cold water or sucking on ice chips can provide relief from thirst without consuming large volumes of liquid.

4.4 Managing Thirst Effectively

Intense, persistent thirst is one of the most challenging symptoms for individuals with DI. While staying hydrated is crucial, managing excessive thirst without overhydrating is key.

1. Strategies for Reducing Thirst Sensation

- **Suck on Sugar-Free Candies or Ice Chips**: This can help reduce the sensation of thirst without significantly adding to fluid intake.
- **Moisten the Mouth**: Rinse your mouth with water and spit it out rather than swallowing to moisten the mouth and trick the brain into feeling quenched.
- **Chew Gum**: Chewing sugar-free gum can stimulate saliva production, reducing the feeling of dryness.

2. Choose Hydration-Aiding Foods

- **Water-Rich Foods**: Foods such as cucumbers, watermelon, and oranges contain high water content and contribute to hydration.

- **Balanced Meals**: Ensure meals include a mix of protein, carbohydrates, and healthy fats to help regulate body hydration and energy.

4.5 Tips for Special Situations
1. Physical Activity

- **Pre-Hydrate and Rehydrate**: Drink water before exercise and replenish fluids lost during physical activity with electrolyte-rich drinks.
- **Hydration During Workouts**: Sip water during exercise rather than gulping large amounts, and use a timer if needed to pace yourself.

2. Travel and Outdoor Activities

- **Prepare Ahead**: When traveling, carry a supply of water and electrolyte solutions. Ensure you know where you can access clean water if traveling to unfamiliar locations.
- **Portable Water Containers**: Use refillable bottles with measurements to track your intake throughout the day.

3. Sick Days

- **Managing Fevers and Illness**: Illness can exacerbate fluid loss. On days when you experience fever, vomiting, or diarrhea, use electrolyte solutions and monitor intake closely.
- **Consult Healthcare Provider**: For significant changes in fluid loss due to illness, consult your healthcare provider for adjusted intake recommendations.

4.6 Common Challenges and Solutions
1. Dealing with Social Situations

- **Planning Ahead**: In social settings, inform hosts or carry water bottles discreetly to manage fluid intake without drawing attention.
- **Communicating with Others**: Educate friends and family about your condition so they can support your needs.

2. Managing Nocturia

- **Limit Fluids Before Bed**: Reduce water intake in the late evening to minimize nighttime urination.
- **Comfort Strategies**: Use nightlights in hallways and bathrooms to make frequent trips to the restroom easier during the night.

Proper hydration is a dynamic process that requires careful attention and adaptation. By implementing these comprehensive strategies, individuals with DI can maintain optimal hydration, manage their symptoms more effectively, and enhance their overall quality of life. Safe water intake, proactive monitoring, and targeted thirst management techniques are essential tools for thriving despite the challenges of DI.

Chapter 5: Eating Right – Dietary Choices for DI Wellness

Diet plays a vital role in managing Diabetes Insipidus (DI), complementing medical treatment and hydration strategies. The right dietary choices can help maintain electrolyte balance, manage thirst, and support overall health. This chapter provides an extensive look at foods to prioritize, hydration-friendly meals, and tips for balancing electrolytes to better manage DI symptoms.

5.1 The Importance of Diet in DI Management

While diet alone cannot replace medical treatments for DI, it plays an essential supportive role. Proper nutrition helps mitigate the risk of dehydration, prevent imbalances in key minerals, and reduce the impact of excessive urination. Strategic food choices can enhance hydration and supply necessary nutrients that aid bodily functions, improving energy levels and overall quality of life.

Key Goals of a DI-Friendly Diet:

- Support hydration and minimize water loss
- Maintain balanced electrolyte levels (sodium, potassium, magnesium)
- Provide sustained energy throughout the day
- Reduce strain on the kidneys and digestive system

5.2 Recommended Foods for DI

Choosing the right foods can help manage hydration and electrolyte levels effectively. Here's a breakdown of beneficial food groups and their roles:

1. Water-Rich Foods Incorporating water-dense foods into your diet can help maintain hydration without the need to drink excessive amounts of liquid.

- **Fruits**: Watermelon, strawberries, cantaloupe, oranges, and grapes
- **Vegetables**: Cucumbers, celery, lettuce, zucchini, and tomatoes
- **Hydration Benefits**: These foods have high water content and are easy to digest, providing a slow release of water into the body and aiding in hydration.

2. Foods High in Electrolytes Maintaining a balance of electrolytes like sodium, potassium, and magnesium is crucial for muscle function, nerve signaling, and preventing dehydration.

- **Sodium-Rich Foods** (in moderation): Pickles, olives, canned soups (low-sodium options when possible), and broths
- **Potassium-Rich Foods**: Bananas, sweet potatoes, spinach, avocados, and apricots
- **Magnesium-Rich Foods**: Almonds, pumpkin seeds, spinach, and whole grains
- **Calcium Sources**: Dairy products, fortified plant-based milk, and leafy greens

3. Protein-Rich Foods Proteins support muscle health and overall bodily repair. Include lean proteins that do not cause excessive thirst or stress on the kidneys.

- **Lean Proteins**: Chicken breast, turkey, fish, tofu, and legumes
- **Dairy Options**: Yogurt and cottage cheese (opt for low-sodium versions)

4. Healthy Carbohydrates Complex carbohydrates provide sustained energy and are often associated with water retention, which can be beneficial for hydration.

- **Whole Grains**: Brown rice, oats, quinoa, and whole wheat pasta
- **Legumes**: Lentils, chickpeas, and black beans
- **Root Vegetables**: Sweet potatoes and carrots

5.3 Hydration-Friendly Meals

Designing meals that are hydration-friendly and nutrient-rich can make managing DI easier. Here are some meal suggestions that balance water content, electrolytes, and essential nutrients:

1. Breakfast Options

- **Fruit and Yogurt Bowl**: Combine water-rich fruits like watermelon and strawberries with yogurt, adding a sprinkle of chia seeds for omega-3s.
- **Oatmeal with Banana and Almonds**: Oats cooked in water or low-sodium plant milk, topped with sliced bananas and almonds for added potassium and magnesium.

2. Lunch Ideas

- **Hydration Salad**: Mix cucumbers, tomatoes, lettuce, celery, and avocado. Dress with a light vinaigrette and add grilled chicken or tofu for protein.
- **Quinoa and Vegetable Bowl**: Quinoa cooked with low-sodium vegetable broth, combined with spinach, sweet potato chunks, and chickpeas.

3. Dinner Dishes

- **Grilled Salmon with Spinach and Brown Rice**: A meal rich in omega-3 fatty acids and potassium. Serve with a side of water-rich steamed vegetables.
- **Chicken and Broccoli Stir-Fry**: Prepared with garlic and a low-sodium soy sauce alternative, served over a small portion of brown rice.

4. Snacks and Light Meals

- **Fruit Smoothie**: Blend water-dense fruits with a handful of spinach and a splash of coconut water for added electrolytes.
- **Trail Mix**: Make a DIY trail mix with unsalted nuts, dried apricots, and pumpkin seeds for a magnesium and potassium boost.
- **Veggie Sticks with Hummus**: Carrot and cucumber sticks paired with hummus for a hydrating, nutrient-dense snack.

5.4 Managing Electrolyte Balance

A significant concern for those with DI is maintaining proper electrolyte levels, as excessive urination can lead to the loss of these vital minerals.

1. Sodium Balance

- **Avoid Excess Sodium**: While sodium is essential for fluid balance, excessive amounts can exacerbate thirst. Stick to moderate levels and avoid processed foods high in sodium.
- **Sodium Replenishment**: When needed, low-sodium broths or sports drinks specifically formulated for hydration can be used to restore sodium levels.

2. Potassium Intake

- **Potassium-Rich Meals**: Include foods like bananas, potatoes, and beans regularly in your diet to maintain potassium levels, as this mineral helps with muscle function and prevents cramping.
- **Symptoms of Low Potassium**: Weakness, fatigue, and muscle cramps are indicators that you may need more potassium.

3. Magnesium for Muscle and Nerve Health

- **Sources of Magnesium**: Spinach, almonds, and pumpkin seeds are excellent sources.
- **Supplementation**: If dietary sources are not enough, consult your healthcare provider about taking a magnesium supplement.

4. Balancing Electrolytes with Hydration Solutions

- **Oral Rehydration Solutions (ORS)**: Use these solutions, especially during periods of illness or high physical activity, to maintain a balance of sodium and potassium.
- **Coconut Water**: This natural beverage is high in potassium and contains natural sugars for energy, making it a good option for rehydration.

5.5 Foods to Limit or Avoid

Some foods and beverages can aggravate symptoms of DI or increase the risk of dehydration. It's essential to be aware of these and limit their intake.

1. Caffeine and Alcohol

- **Diuretic Effect**: Both caffeine and alcohol can increase urine production and lead to greater fluid loss.
- **Moderation**: If consumed, do so in moderation and ensure increased water intake to counteract their dehydrating effects.

2. High-Sodium Processed Foods

- **Fast Foods and Packaged Snacks**: Items such as chips, processed meats, and instant noodles contain high sodium levels that can increase thirst.

- **Healthier Alternatives**: Opt for low-sodium versions or make homemade versions with controlled salt content.

3. Sugary Beverages

- **Sodas and Sweetened Drinks**: These do not contribute to proper hydration and can lead to spikes in blood sugar, potentially exacerbating thirst.
- **Better Choices**: Stick to water, herbal teas, or diluted fruit juices without added sugars.

5.6 Special Considerations and Tips
1. Managing Meals During Social Gatherings

- **Plan Ahead**: If attending an event or dining out, review the menu beforehand and choose water-rich, low-sodium options.
- **Stay Hydrated**: Drink a glass of water before meals to prevent overeating and help with digestion.

2. Preparing Meals in Advance

- **Meal Prep for Convenience**: Prepare hydration-friendly meals in advance to have nutrient-rich options on hand when time is limited.
- **Balanced Containers**: Store pre-made salads, grain bowls, and hydration-rich snacks in containers that make them easy to grab and go.

3. Listen to Your Body

- **Adjust Diet as Needed**: Individual needs may vary, so pay attention to how your body responds to different foods and adjust your diet accordingly.

- **Consult a Dietitian**: Work with a dietitian familiar with DI to create a personalized meal plan that supports your overall health and hydration goals.

Adopting a diet that aligns with the unique needs of DI can help manage symptoms, support hydration, and improve overall well-being. By prioritizing water-rich, nutrient-dense foods and carefully balancing electrolyte intake, individuals with DI can enhance their quality of life and reduce the impact of excessive fluid loss.

Chapter 6: Emergency Essentials – Preparing for the Unexpected

For individuals living with Diabetes Insipidus (DI), being prepared for unexpected situations is essential to ensure safety and maintain health during emergencies. This chapter provides an in-depth guide to creating a comprehensive emergency kit, ensuring access to backup hydration, and compiling important medical contacts and information. Preparedness can help manage DI effectively in various scenarios, from power outages and natural disasters to travel and unforeseen medical situations.

6.1 The Importance of an Emergency Kit

An emergency kit tailored to the specific needs of someone with DI serves as a vital safety net. It helps maintain health and hydration when regular access to medication, clean water, or healthcare facilities may be disrupted.

Why an Emergency Kit is Essential:

- **Immediate Access**: Quick access to necessary medications and supplies can prevent dangerous dehydration or an electrolyte imbalance.
- **Peace of Mind**: Knowing you have a prepared kit can reduce anxiety about facing unexpected situations.
- **Portability**: A well-organized kit can be grabbed quickly and taken anywhere, ensuring preparedness even during an evacuation or sudden relocation.

6.2 Core Components of a DI Emergency Kit

A well-rounded emergency kit for someone with DI should include essential medications, hydration aids, and other items that support health and safety. Below is a comprehensive breakdown of what to include:

1. Medications and Medical Supplies

- **Primary Medications**: Ensure an adequate supply of prescribed medications, such as desmopressin (DDAVP), thiazide diuretics, or any other medications used to manage DI. Store these in original packaging with clear labels and include dosage instructions.
- **Backup Medications**: Have an extra supply of medication stored separately in case the primary stock is damaged or runs out. Ensure these are within their expiration date.
- **Medication Cooler**: For medications that need to be kept cool (e.g., injectable desmopressin), include an insulated cooler bag with ice packs to maintain the proper temperature.
- **Prescription Copies**: Include copies of all current prescriptions, both in paper form and saved digitally on a secure USB drive or a smartphone app.
- **Pill Organizer**: A weekly pill organizer can help keep track of daily dosages during chaotic situations.

2. Hydration and Electrolyte Solutions

- **Bottled Water**: Keep several liters of bottled water in the kit. Choose sealed, commercially prepared water bottles with long shelf lives.

- **Oral Rehydration Solutions (ORS)**: Include packets of ORS powder that can be mixed with water to replenish electrolytes quickly.
- **Electrolyte Tablets**: Compact and easy to carry, electrolyte tablets can be dissolved in water to provide a quick boost of essential minerals.
- **Hydration-Friendly Foods**: Canned or sealed fruit cups and snacks like electrolyte-rich energy bars can provide hydration and nutrition.

3. Medical Information Packet

- **Emergency Medical Information Card**: Include a card with your name, condition (DI), key symptoms, current medications, and any known allergies. This should be easy to access for first responders.
- **Contact List**: Compile a list of important medical contacts, including your primary care physician, endocrinologist, and pharmacy. Also include the contact information for trusted family members or friends.
- **Medical Records**: Keep copies of recent lab results and a summary of your medical history that can be shared with healthcare providers if needed.
- **Insurance Information**: Include copies of health insurance cards and any relevant policy information.

4. First Aid Supplies

- **Basic First Aid Kit**: Pack bandages, antiseptic wipes, gauze, adhesive tape, and pain relievers.
- **Thermometer**: A digital thermometer to monitor body temperature, which can help identify fever or illness that may exacerbate DI symptoms.

- **Blood Pressure Monitor**: For individuals prone to blood pressure fluctuations, a compact monitor can provide valuable information during stressful situations.

6.3 Additional Emergency Preparedness Tips
1. Organize and Label the Kit

- **Clear Labeling**: Clearly label all containers and pouches in the kit so that anyone (even someone unfamiliar with DI) can understand its contents.
- **Waterproof Containers**: Store medications and medical documents in waterproof pouches to protect them from damage in wet conditions.

2. Accessibility and Portability

- **Keep the Kit Within Reach**: Store the emergency kit in an easily accessible location, such as near an exit or in your car, so it can be grabbed quickly in an emergency.
- **Portable Bag or Backpack**: Use a sturdy, waterproof bag or backpack to house the kit, making it easy to carry during evacuations.

3. Maintain the Kit Regularly

- **Check Expiration Dates**: Regularly review the contents of the kit to ensure medications, water, and food items are not expired. Replace items as needed.
- **Seasonal Adjustments**: Update the kit seasonally with relevant items, such as a cooling towel for hot weather or hand warmers for cold conditions.

4. Include Comfort Items

- **Blankets and Clothing**: Add a lightweight blanket or extra clothing for comfort in case of prolonged stays outside the home.
- **Flashlight and Batteries**: Pack a battery-operated or hand-crank flashlight with spare batteries.
- **Power Bank for Devices**: Include a fully charged power bank to keep your phone and other electronics powered during an outage.

6.4 Backup Hydration Strategies

When regular water access is disrupted, it's crucial to have backup plans for maintaining hydration:

1. Water Purification Tools

- **Portable Water Filter**: Include a compact, portable water filter or water purification straw that can make most freshwater sources safe to drink.
- **Water Purification Tablets**: These tablets can be used to treat water, making it potable in emergencies where clean water is not available.
- **Collapsible Water Containers**: These are ideal for storing water collected from external sources.

2. Storing Water at Home

- **Long-Term Water Storage**: For those in disaster-prone areas, consider storing larger water containers at home with treatment to prevent bacterial growth.

- **Labeling**: Clearly label all water containers with the date of storage to ensure freshness.

6.5 Essential Medical Contacts and Information

Compiling a comprehensive list of medical contacts and crucial health information can be life-saving during an emergency:

1. Medical Contacts

- **Primary Care Physician and Specialists**: Include names, phone numbers, and email addresses of your primary care doctor, endocrinologist, and nephrologist.
- **Pharmacy Contact**: List the name and number of your preferred pharmacy and any backup pharmacies.
- **Emergency Medical Services**: Note the contact information for local emergency services and hospitals familiar with treating rare conditions like DI.

2. Family and Caregiver Information

- **Emergency Contacts**: List family members, close friends, or caregivers who understand your medical needs and can assist in an emergency.
- **Consent to Treat**: Include a statement giving consent for a trusted individual to authorize medical treatment if you are unable to do so.

3. Local and National Resources

- **Support Organizations**: Include contact information for support organizations such as DI-specific advocacy groups or general chronic illness support networks.

- **Government Services**: List local emergency management services, Red Cross contacts, and other agencies that provide assistance during emergencies.

6.6 Practice and Preparation
1. Emergency Drills

- **Run Drills**: Periodically practice accessing and using your emergency kit to ensure you're familiar with its contents.
- **Family Involvement**: If you live with others, make sure they know where the kit is stored and how to use it.

2. Travel Preparation

- **Portable Kit for Travel**: When traveling, create a compact version of your emergency kit that includes essential items such as medications, a water purification straw, and medical information.
- **Check Local Resources**: Research the healthcare facilities and emergency services available at your destination.

3. Communication Plan

- **Share Your Plan**: Let family and emergency contacts know your plan and where to find your emergency kit.
- **Alert Apps**: Consider using smartphone apps that can send alerts to emergency contacts if you need help.

Preparing for emergencies when you have DI involves careful planning and attention to detail. By assembling a well-stocked emergency kit, ensuring access to backup hydration, and having vital medical information readily available, you can protect your health and well-being in unexpected situations. Taking proactive steps today means being ready for whatever tomorrow may bring.

Chapter 7: Managing DI at Work and School – Tips for Daily Life

Living with Diabetes Insipidus (DI) presents unique challenges that can impact your day-to-day life, especially in structured environments like the workplace or school. Frequent bathroom breaks, maintaining hydration, and potential fatigue can disrupt routines if not managed proactively. This chapter provides detailed strategies for explaining your condition to employers, teachers, and colleagues while offering practical advice for managing symptoms discreetly and effectively.

7.1 How to Explain DI to Employers, Teachers, and Colleagues

Disclosing your condition can feel daunting, but open communication often leads to better understanding and necessary accommodations. Here's how to navigate those conversations:

1. Deciding When and Who to Tell

- **Evaluate the Need**: If your DI significantly impacts your daily routine, such as needing frequent restroom breaks or adhering to a strict hydration schedule, it's wise to inform your employer, supervisor, or school administrators.
- **Choose Key Individuals**: Start with those who can provide accommodations, such as HR representatives, supervisors, teachers, or school counselors. This ensures that your needs are met without oversharing with unnecessary contacts.

2. Preparing for the Conversation

- **Understand Your Rights**: Familiarize yourself with local laws and workplace policies, such as the Americans with Disabilities Act (ADA) in the U.S., which mandates reasonable accommodations for employees with medical conditions.
- **Plan Your Explanation**: Keep your description straightforward. Emphasize how DI affects your daily activities and the simple measures that can be taken to accommodate your needs.

- **Bring Documentation**: Have medical documentation or a letter from your doctor that outlines your condition and the adjustments needed, such as frequent restroom breaks or access to water.

Sample Script for Explaining DI: *"I have a condition called Diabetes Insipidus, which affects my body's ability to balance water. This means I need to stay hydrated and may require more frequent bathroom breaks. With a few adjustments, I can effectively manage my responsibilities without any issues."*

3. Emphasizing Management and Reliability

- **Highlight Your Adaptability**: Reassure your employer or teacher that you have methods to manage your condition, such as scheduled hydration, medication adherence, and discreet symptom management.
- **Discuss Solutions**: Offer solutions, like flexible break times or sitting near the restroom, to make accommodating your needs seamless.

7.2 Managing Symptoms Discreetly

Maintaining discretion while managing your DI symptoms helps you stay comfortable and productive without unnecessary attention. Below are some strategies to integrate into your daily routine:

1. Hydration Management

- **Keep a Water Bottle Handy**: Use a refillable, discreet water bottle that can be kept at your desk or workstation. Choose a design that fits into your environment to avoid drawing attention.
- **Set Drinking Timelines**: Sip water throughout the day during natural breaks, like between classes or meetings, to maintain hydration without needing sudden, large intakes.

- **Use Electrolyte Solutions**: Keep single-serve electrolyte packets in your bag or drawer to mix with water as needed. This supports hydration while maintaining electrolyte balance.

2. Scheduling Bathroom Breaks

- **Plan Breaks Wisely**: If your schedule allows, coordinate bathroom visits during set times, such as before or after meetings or between classes, to avoid interruptions.
- **Strategic Seating**: Choose a seat near the exit when in meetings, classrooms, or auditoriums. This minimizes disruption if you need to leave suddenly.
- **Communicate Privately**: Let your supervisor or teacher know that you may need to leave occasionally. Doing this discreetly ensures understanding without drawing attention.

3. Medication Adherence

- **Accessible Medications**: Keep medications like desmopressin or other prescribed treatments in an easy-to-access but discreet container, such as a small pillbox or pouch.
- **Silent Reminders**: Set silent alarms or smartphone notifications to remind you when to take your medication, ensuring you stay on track without interruptions.

4. Handling Fatigue

- **Take Mini-Breaks**: Short breaks to rest your eyes or stretch can help combat fatigue during long work or school hours. Use these breaks for light stretching or a few minutes of quiet rest.
- **Snack Smartly**: Keep energy-boosting, non-thirst-provoking snacks on hand, such as nuts, yogurt, or fresh fruit, to maintain energy without increasing thirst.

7.3 Building a Supportive Environment

A supportive environment at work or school can greatly enhance your ability to manage DI effectively. Here's how to foster understanding and cooperation:

1. Educate Trusted Individuals

- **Selective Sharing**: Inform close colleagues or classmates who you trust and who can assist if necessary. Sharing a basic understanding of your condition helps them provide support when needed.
- **Keep it Simple**: Use plain language to explain DI, emphasizing its management and minimal impact on daily activities with the right accommodations.

2. Utilize Resources

- **Engage with HR or School Services**: Discuss potential accommodations, such as flexible breaks, modified workstations, or access to water and restrooms. Ensure these are documented for your protection.
- **504 Plans and IEPs for Students**: For students, schools may offer formal plans that ensure accommodations like extended time for tests or flexible scheduling for restroom use.

3. Build a Support Network

- **Peer Support**: Identify coworkers or classmates who understand your situation and can step in or support you when needed.
- **Join or Advocate for Employee Resource Groups (ERGs)**: If your workplace or school has ERGs focused on health and wellness, participate in them. If not, consider advocating for one that can support individuals with chronic conditions.

7.4 Stress Management and DI

Stress can exacerbate DI symptoms and make managing your condition more difficult. Implementing stress management practices can improve both your mental and physical well-being.

1. Time Management Techniques

- **Plan Ahead**: Prioritize tasks to avoid last-minute stress, which can increase your need for hydration and exacerbate fatigue.
- **Flexible Scheduling**: Work with your employer or school to create a schedule that accommodates your energy levels and symptom management.

2. Mindfulness Practices

- **Breathing Exercises**: Short, deep breathing exercises can help reduce stress and promote focus during the day.
- **Mindful Breaks**: Take moments throughout the day to pause, relax, and reset your mind. This can be done with short guided meditations or quiet time away from your desk or classroom.

3. Support Services

- **Counseling and Therapy**: Access counseling services at work or school for additional support in managing stress and adapting to challenges.
- **Employee Assistance Programs (EAPs)**: Check if your workplace offers EAPs, which can provide counseling and other resources to help manage stress.

7.5 Handling Business Travel or School Excursions

Work trips or school outings can disrupt routines and add stress. Preparation is key to managing DI in these situations:

1. Prepare a Portable Kit

- **Medication Case**: Carry a travel-sized case with enough medication for the duration of your trip, plus a backup supply.
- **Travel Water Bottle**: Pack a lightweight, refillable water bottle to ensure access to water at all times.
- **Snacks and Electrolytes**: Include energy-boosting snacks and packets of ORS or electrolyte tablets.

2. Plan for Accessibility

- **Scout Facilities**: Research available restrooms and water stations at your destination beforehand.
- **Notify Trip Coordinators**: Inform relevant trip organizers about your condition and the need for possible adjustments.

3. Keep Essential Documents

- **Medical ID**: Carry a medical ID card or bracelet that indicates your DI diagnosis and emergency contact information.
- **Insurance and Emergency Contacts**: Have copies of insurance details and a list of emergency contacts on hand.

7.6 Navigating Social Situations

Managing DI in social settings at work or school requires subtle strategies to avoid discomfort or attention:

1. Handling Questions

- **Simple Explanations**: Be prepared with a brief explanation like, "I have a condition that requires me to stay hydrated and take regular breaks." This helps others understand without delving into detailed medical information.
- **Redirect the Conversation**: Shift focus back to the topic at hand after your brief explanation to keep the conversation light.

2. Setting Boundaries

- **Respect Personal Limits**: Recognize when an activity or situation may not be suitable for your condition and politely decline or suggest an alternative.
- **Speak Up When Needed**: If a meeting or event is prolonged and becomes uncomfortable due to your DI needs, request a brief pause or step out as required.

7.7 Key Takeaways for Managing DI in Daily Life

Successfully managing DI at work or school involves planning, communication, and self-awareness. With open discussions, discreet symptom management, and a supportive environment, you can balance your responsibilities and maintain your health. Implementing the strategies outlined in this chapter can empower you to thrive in daily life while effectively managing your DI symptoms.

Chapter 8: Staying Active Safely – Exercise and Physical Health

Physical activity is a crucial component of overall well-being, and for individuals with Diabetes Insipidus (DI), staying active can support cardiovascular health, boost energy levels, and enhance mental health. However, due to the nature of DI, there are specific challenges related to exercise, such as managing hydration and preventing dehydration. This chapter will provide detailed guidance on safe exercise practices, hydration strategies during workouts, and how to stay active without exacerbating DI symptoms.

8.1 Benefits of Exercise for Individuals with DI

Regular physical activity offers numerous benefits that can positively impact those with DI:

- **Improved Cardiovascular Health**: Exercise strengthens the heart and improves circulation, which can enhance energy levels and overall stamina.
- **Weight Management**: Physical activity helps maintain a healthy weight, which can reduce the strain on the body and improve overall health.
- **Enhanced Mood and Stress Reduction**: Exercise releases endorphins, which promote a positive mood and reduce stress. This can be particularly beneficial as stress can exacerbate DI symptoms.
- **Increased Muscle Strength and Bone Density**: Weight-bearing exercises can support bone health and prevent muscle loss.

8.2 Challenges of Exercising with DI

Individuals with DI face unique challenges when it comes to staying active:

- **Dehydration Risks**: Due to the body's inability to retain water effectively, the risk of dehydration during exercise is higher.
- **Electrolyte Imbalance**: Excessive sweating and frequent urination can lead to a loss of vital electrolytes, affecting muscle function and overall health.
- **Fatigue**: The need to manage hydration and frequent bathroom breaks can lead to exercise fatigue or disrupt workout routines.

Understanding and addressing these challenges is key to developing a safe and effective exercise plan.

8.3 Preparing for Exercise

Proper preparation helps ensure a safe and effective workout. Here are essential pre-exercise practices to follow:

1. Hydrate Beforehand

- **Pre-Hydration**: Drink water or an electrolyte solution 30–60 minutes before starting your exercise session. This helps build a hydration reserve to counter water loss during physical activity.
- **Balanced Intake**: Avoid overhydrating before a workout, as this can dilute sodium levels and lead to hyponatremia. Aim for moderate hydration that is consistent with your body's needs.

2. Choose the Right Time

- **Exercise in Cooler Hours**: Opt for early morning or late evening workouts to avoid excessive heat and sweating, which can lead to rapid fluid loss.

- **Monitor Weather Conditions**: High temperatures and humidity can exacerbate water loss, so adjust your workout duration and intensity accordingly.

3. Wear Appropriate Clothing

- **Breathable Fabric**: Choose lightweight, moisture-wicking clothing that helps keep your body cool and minimizes excessive sweating.
- **Comfortable Fit**: Opt for loose clothing that allows freedom of movement and air circulation.

4. Plan Your Routine

- **Low-Impact Options**: Start with low- to moderate-impact exercises such as walking, cycling, swimming, or yoga. These activities allow for a gradual increase in intensity without overwhelming the body.
- **Strength Training**: Incorporate strength training exercises with light weights or resistance bands to build muscle without excessive exertion.

8.4 Safe Practices During Exercise

Staying safe while exercising with DI involves carefully monitoring your hydration status, energy levels, and environmental conditions.

1. Monitor Hydration

- **Hydrate Consistently**: Take sips of water throughout your workout instead of large gulps to prevent overhydration and maintain steady hydration.
- **Electrolyte Solutions**: Incorporate drinks that contain electrolytes to replenish lost minerals, especially during longer or

more intense workouts. Choose solutions with a balanced mix of sodium, potassium, and magnesium.

- **Water Bottles**: Carry a reusable water bottle with clear volume markers to track how much water you are consuming during your exercise session.

2. Pay Attention to Your Body

- **Recognize Early Signs of Dehydration**: Symptoms such as dizziness, dry mouth, and a rapid heartbeat indicate dehydration. Stop exercising immediately and rehydrate if these symptoms occur.
- **Monitor Fatigue Levels**: If you feel unusually fatigued, light-headed, or weak, pause your workout, take a break, and reassess your hydration status.

3. Take Breaks

- **Scheduled Rest Periods**: Include short breaks during your workout to rest and drink water. This helps prevent overexertion and gives your body time to recover.
- **Cooling Techniques**: Use a cooling towel or splash cool water on your face and neck during breaks to help regulate your body temperature.

4. Avoid High-Intensity Workouts in Extreme Conditions

- **Limit High-Intensity Sessions**: While high-intensity interval training (HIIT) and vigorous exercise can be beneficial, they may not be suitable for everyone with DI, especially in hot and humid environments.
- **Opt for Indoor Workouts**: During extreme weather conditions, opt for indoor exercises such as treadmill walking, station-

ary cycling, or light aerobics in a temperature-controlled environment.

8.5 Hydration Strategies During Workouts

Managing hydration is the most critical aspect of exercising with DI. Follow these strategies to maintain proper hydration:

1. Drink Smart

- **Small, Regular Sips**: Sip water regularly throughout your workout rather than waiting until you feel thirsty. This prevents sudden dehydration and helps maintain fluid levels.
- **Include Electrolytes**: Supplement your hydration with electrolyte-infused water or tablets that dissolve in water. This ensures that you replenish not only water but also essential minerals lost through sweat.

2. Listen to Your Thirst Cues

- **Avoid Overhydration**: Drinking too much water too quickly can dilute sodium levels in your blood, leading to hyponatremia. Listen to your body's cues and balance water intake with electrolytes.
- **Monitor Urine Color Post-Workout**: After exercising, check the color of your urine as an indicator of hydration status. Light yellow is typically a sign of adequate hydration, while darker urine may indicate the need for more fluids.

3. Carry Rehydration Essentials

- **ORS Packets**: Oral rehydration solution (ORS) packets can be easily added to water for quick electrolyte replenishment during or after a workout.

- **Portable Electrolyte Tablets**: Keep electrolyte tablets in your gym bag to dissolve in your water bottle when needed.

8.6 Managing Post-Exercise Recovery

Recovery is an important part of maintaining a balanced exercise routine for individuals with DI:

1. Rehydrate Properly

- **Post-Workout Hydration**: Continue hydrating with water and electrolyte solutions after exercise to replace fluids lost during your session.
- **Balanced Rehydration**: Drink fluids at a moderate pace over an hour or two to avoid overwhelming your kidneys.

2. Cool Down and Stretch

- **Stretching Routine**: Include light stretching after your work-out to relax your muscles, reduce soreness, and prevent stiffness.
- **Breathing Exercises**: Incorporate deep breathing exercises to regulate your heart rate and promote a sense of calm.

3. Refuel with Nutrient-Dense Foods

- **Electrolyte-Rich Snacks**: Snack on foods high in potassium, such as bananas or dried apricots, and foods rich in magnesium, like almonds, to replenish lost minerals.
- **Balanced Meals**: Eat a balanced meal that includes lean protein, complex carbohydrates, and healthy fats to aid muscle recovery and sustain energy levels.

4. Monitor Post-Exercise Symptoms

- **Be Alert to Signs of Imbalance**: Watch for symptoms such as muscle cramps, fatigue, or prolonged dizziness after exercise, which could indicate electrolyte imbalances or dehydration.
- **Communicate with Your Doctor**: If post-exercise symptoms persist or worsen, consult your healthcare provider for tailored advice.

8.7 Adapting Exercise for Different Settings

Staying active can take place in various environments. Here's how to adapt exercise for different settings:

1. At Home

- **Home Workouts**: Use online videos or apps for guided yoga, pilates, or low-impact cardio sessions.
- **Create a Safe Space**: Ensure your home workout area is well-ventilated and set up with water and electrolyte drinks within reach.

2. At the Gym

- **Choose Equipment Wisely**: Opt for machines that allow you to monitor intensity, such as treadmills or stationary bikes with heart rate monitors.
- **Stay Near Hydration Stations**: Position yourself near water fountains or bring your own water to ensure easy access during your workout.

3. Outdoor Activities

- **Stay Cool**: Wear a hat and sunscreen, and choose shaded paths for outdoor activities like jogging or hiking.
- **Prepare for Longer Outings**: Carry a hydration pack or water belt that holds sufficient water and electrolyte solutions.

8.8 When to Consult Your Doctor

Before starting any new exercise routine, it's essential to consult your doctor, especially if you have DI:

1. Get Medical Clearance

- **Personalized Recommendations**: Your doctor can suggest the best types of exercises based on your health status and specific DI needs.
- **Monitor Initial Responses**: Work with your doctor to monitor how your body responds to exercise and adjust your routine accordingly.

2. Report Unusual Symptoms

- **Post-Exercise Reactions**: If you experience unusual symptoms such as severe fatigue, persistent dizziness, or rapid heart rate changes during or after exercise, seek medical advice.
- **Adjustments to Treatment**: Your doctor may recommend changes to your hydration plan or medication to better align with your exercise routine.

Staying active with Diabetes Insipidus requires careful preparation, hydration strategies, and the ability to recognize your body's limits.

With the right approach, exercise can be an enjoyable and beneficial part of managing DI, enhancing physical health and overall well-being.

Chapter 9: DI on the Go – Traveling with Confidence

Traveling can be both an exciting and daunting prospect for individuals with Diabetes Insipidus (DI). Ensuring consistent access to water, maintaining medication schedules, and staying prepared for unexpected situations are crucial for a safe and enjoyable trip. This chapter provides a comprehensive guide for planning and managing DI while traveling, covering hydration strategies, medication management, and essential travel preparations.

9.1 Pre-Travel Planning

Thorough preparation is the key to a successful trip for those with DI. Taking proactive measures before leaving can prevent complications and ensure you are ready for any scenario.

1. Research Your Destination

- **Access to Water**: Confirm that your destination has reliable access to clean drinking water. Research local stores, water refill stations, and pharmacies.
- **Climate Considerations**: Understand the climate at your destination. Hot and humid weather can increase the risk of dehydration, while cold environments may require different hydration strategies.
- **Medical Facilities**: Identify the nearest hospitals, clinics, and pharmacies that can assist in case of a medical emergency.

2. Create a Travel Checklist

- **Medications**: Ensure you pack all required medications, including desmopressin (DDAVP) and any other prescribed treatments. Include extra doses in case of delays or lost luggage.
- **Hydration Essentials**: Pack a sufficient number of water bottles, electrolyte solutions, and portable water filters.

- **Medical Information**: Carry a medical ID card that explains your condition, outlines your medication, and lists emergency contacts.

3. Notify Your Travel Companions

- **Educate Travel Partners**: Inform your travel companions about your condition and any assistance you might need. This helps them support you if you face any challenges.
- **Share Emergency Plans**: Ensure at least one travel partner knows what to do in case of an emergency, including how to help you access medical care or provide fluids and medication.

9.2 Packing for Travel

A well-prepared travel kit can make managing DI much easier. Pack strategically to ensure you have everything needed for hydration, medication, and comfort.

1. Essential Medication Kit

- **Medications in Original Packaging**: Keep medications in their original containers with prescription labels for easy identification by airport security or customs officials.
- **Backup Supplies**: Bring more medication than you expect to need. Store a backup supply in a separate bag in case one gets lost or damaged.
- **Portable Medication Cooler**: If your medication requires refrigeration, pack it in a portable cooler bag with ice packs to maintain the correct temperature during transit.

2. Hydration Tools

- **Reusable Water Bottles**: Bring a durable, refillable water bottle with volume markers to track your fluid intake. Collapsible bottles can save space.
- **Electrolyte Packets and Tablets**: Carry single-serve electrolyte powder or tablets to add to water for quick hydration.
- **Portable Water Filters**: A compact water filtration system or purification tablets can help ensure safe drinking water if bottled water isn't available.

3. Comfort and Support Items

- **Cooling Towels**: For travel in warm climates, cooling towels can help regulate your body temperature and reduce the need for excessive hydration.
- **Small Snacks**: Pack snacks like dried fruit, nuts, or energy bars that provide nutrients without significantly increasing thirst.
- **Emergency Contacts and Information**: Keep a printed list of important contacts, such as your doctor, pharmacy, and emergency contacts, in your travel kit.

9.3 Navigating Airports and Security

Airport travel involves unique challenges, such as navigating security checks and dealing with potential delays. Planning ahead can help you manage these obstacles with confidence.

1. Communicating with Security Personnel

- **Declare Medical Needs**: Inform security personnel that you have a medical condition and may need to carry medications, liquids, or medical devices.
- **Present Documentation**: Provide a doctor's note or medical certificate that explains your condition and lists the medications you need to carry.
- **Medication Inspection**: Be prepared for medications and liquid containers to be inspected. Ensure they are in transparent, labeled bags to expedite the process.

2. Managing Hydration During Flights

- **Stay Hydrated**: Airplane cabins can be dehydrating, so drink water regularly. Bring your own water bottle and ask flight attendants for refills as needed.
- **Avoid Overhydration**: Balance water intake with electrolyte solutions to prevent hyponatremia. Take small, consistent sips instead of drinking large amounts at once.
- **Restroom Access**: Choose an aisle seat for easier restroom access during long flights.

3. Handling Layovers and Delays

- **Plan for Extra Water and Snacks**: Pack enough water and snacks to last through any unexpected delays.
- **Use Airport Amenities**: Identify water refill stations and restrooms in advance to stay comfortable during layovers.

9.4 Managing DI at Your Destination

Upon arrival, maintaining your routine and ensuring access to necessities are critical for managing DI effectively.

1. Establishing a Hydration Routine

- **Set Hydration Timers**: Use phone alarms or reminders to maintain a consistent hydration schedule.
- **Know Your Environment**: Adapt your water intake based on local temperature and humidity. For hotter climates, increase your intake and take more frequent hydration breaks.

2. Safe Drinking Water Practices

- **Stick to Bottled Water**: In areas with questionable water quality, use bottled water for drinking and brushing your teeth.
- **Use Water Purifiers**: If bottled water isn't available, rely on water purification tablets or portable filters to make tap water safe to drink.

3. Managing Medication

- **Secure Storage**: Store medications in a cool, dry place. If your accommodations don't have a refrigerator and you need one, consider requesting one or using an insulated cooler with ice packs.
- **Stay on Schedule**: Adjust medication schedules based on time zone changes, ensuring you don't miss a dose or take it at the wrong time.

4. Handling Activities and Excursions

- **Plan Restroom Access**: Before joining tours, hikes, or excursions, confirm that restrooms will be available.
- **Bring a Hydration Pack**: For longer activities, use a hydration backpack or belt to carry water and electrolytes comfortably.
- **Prepare for Breaks**: Inform guides or group leaders about your condition so that they can plan breaks as needed.

9.5 Staying Prepared for Emergencies

Traveling can sometimes lead to unexpected situations. Being prepared can make all the difference in managing DI safely.

1. Emergency Hydration Solutions

- **Carry ORS Packets**: Pack oral rehydration solution packets in your day bag for quick rehydration during emergencies.
- **Hydration Strategies**: If water is scarce, use electrolyte drinks to stretch your fluid intake and maintain essential electrolyte balance.

2. Access to Medical Help

- **Identify Local Medical Facilities**: Know the location and contact information for the nearest medical facilities and pharmacies.
- **Medical Translation**: If traveling to a non-English-speaking country, carry translated phrases related to your condition and treatment needs.

3. Medical Identification

- **Wear a Medical Alert**: A medical ID bracelet or necklace that explains your condition and states any critical information (e.g., "Diabetes Insipidus – Needs Hydration and Medication") can be life-saving in emergencies.

- **Smartphone Medical ID**: Set up the emergency medical ID function on your smartphone so that first responders can access vital health information even if your phone is locked.

9.6 Tips for Different Types of Travel
1. Road Trips

- **Plan Hydration Stops**: Map out rest stops and gas stations where you can refill water bottles and use the restroom.
- **Cooler with Hydration Supplies**: Keep a cooler stocked with water bottles and electrolyte drinks for easy access during the drive.

2. International Travel

- **Check Medication Regulations**: Research the regulations for carrying medications into your destination country and bring documentation if needed.
- **Time Zone Adjustments**: Gradually adjust your hydration and medication schedule to align with the new time zone before your trip.

3. Outdoor Adventures

- **Stay Equipped**: Pack extra water, a portable water filter, and ORS packets when heading into nature.
- **Communicate with Guides**: Let hiking or tour guides know about your condition and your need for frequent hydration and bathroom breaks.

9.7 After Travel: Recovery and Reassessment

Returning from a trip provides an opportunity to assess how well your travel plan worked and make adjustments for future journeys.

1. Review Hydration and Medication Management

- **Evaluate Your Routine**: Reflect on what worked well and what could be improved in terms of hydration, medication, and symptom management during your trip.
- **Rehydrate Thoroughly**: Replenish fluids and electrolytes if you experienced any dehydration during travel.

2. Update Your Travel Kit

- **Restock Supplies**: Replace any medications, ORS packets, or snacks that were used during the trip.
- **Make Notes**: Write down any observations or lessons learned to refine your travel strategy for next time.

3. Share Experiences

- **Communicate with Your Doctor**: Discuss your travel experiences with your healthcare provider to get advice or adjustments for future trips.
- **Connect with DI Communities**: Share tips or gain insights from other individuals with DI through support groups or online forums.

Traveling with Diabetes Insipidus is entirely manageable with careful planning, strategic hydration, and attention to medication management. By following the guidelines and tips provided in this chapter, you can explore new places, enjoy diverse experiences, and travel with confidence while effectively managing your condition.

Chapter 10: Navigating Finances – Insurance and Cost Management

Managing Diabetes Insipidus (DI) comes with its own set of financial challenges, from securing the right insurance coverage to managing the costs of medications and treatment. Navigating the complexities of health insurance, understanding available financial assistance, and adopting effective cost management strategies can significantly alleviate the financial burden. This chapter provides a comprehensive guide to managing the financial aspects of DI, including navigating insurance, securing financial aid, and tips for managing treatment expenses.

10.1 Understanding Health Insurance for DI

Health insurance plays a crucial role in managing DI, covering the costs of doctor visits, medications, diagnostic tests, and emergency treatments. Here's how to make the most of your health insurance plan:

1. Evaluating Your Insurance Coverage

- **Review Your Policy**: Carefully review your current health insurance policy to ensure it covers DI-related expenses such as specialist visits, prescribed medications (e.g., desmopressin), and lab tests.
- **Check the Formulary**: Confirm whether your medications are included in the insurance company's list of covered drugs (formulary). Different plans may categorize drugs into tiers that determine the cost you'll pay out of pocket.
- **In-Network vs. Out-of-Network**: Use healthcare providers and pharmacies that are in your insurance network to minimize costs. Out-of-network care can result in higher expenses or limited coverage.

2. Understanding Different Types of Plans

- **Health Maintenance Organization (HMO)**: Typically requires using healthcare providers within a specific network and obtaining referrals for specialist visits. HMOs can offer lower premiums but may be more restrictive.
- **Preferred Provider Organization (PPO)**: Offers more flexibility in choosing healthcare providers, including specialists, without needing referrals. PPOs usually come with higher premiums but provide more freedom.
- **High-Deductible Health Plan (HDHP)**: Has lower monthly premiums but higher out-of-pocket costs until the deductible is met. It can be paired with a Health Savings Account (HSA) for tax-advantaged savings.
- **Medicare and Medicaid**: If eligible, these government programs can help cover DI expenses. Medicare typically covers people over 65 or with certain disabilities, while Medicaid is income-based and varies by state.

3. Insurance Terminology to Know

- **Premium**: The amount you pay monthly or annually for insurance coverage.
- **Deductible**: The amount you need to pay out of pocket for medical expenses before your insurance starts covering costs.
- **Co-payment (Co-pay)**: A fixed fee you pay for specific services, such as doctor visits or prescriptions.
- **Coinsurance**: The percentage of medical costs you share with your insurance after meeting your deductible.

10.2 Tips for Maximizing Insurance Benefits

To minimize your out-of-pocket expenses and maximize your insurance benefits, consider the following tips:

1. Use Generic Medications

- **Request Generics**: If available, ask your doctor if a generic version of your prescribed medication, such as desmopressin, can be substituted. Generic drugs are often more affordable and covered by insurance.
- **Compare Prices**: Even with insurance, prices can vary between pharmacies. Use prescription discount programs or apps to find the best price for your medication.

2. Review Benefits Annually

- **Annual Plan Review**: Insurance benefits and coverage details can change each year. Review your plan annually to ensure it still meets your needs, and compare options during open enrollment periods.
- **Plan Adjustments**: If your current plan doesn't provide adequate coverage for your DI treatment, consider switching to a plan that offers better prescription coverage or lower deductibles.

3. Prior Authorization and Appeals

- **Obtain Prior Authorization**: Some medications, especially higher-cost ones, may require prior authorization from your insurance company. Work with your doctor to complete this process to ensure coverage.

- **Appeal Denials**: If your insurance denies coverage for a necessary treatment or medication, file an appeal with supporting documentation from your doctor.

4. Keep Track of Medical Expenses

- **Maintain Records**: Keep detailed records of all medical expenses, including doctor visits, prescription receipts, and insurance claim statements. This documentation can be useful when filing appeals or seeking reimbursement.
- **Use an HSA or FSA**: If you have access to a Health Savings Account (HSA) or Flexible Spending Account (FSA), use it to pay for out-of-pocket medical expenses with pre-tax dollars, reducing your taxable income.

10.3 Managing Treatment Costs

Even with insurance, the costs associated with managing DI can add up. Here are some strategies to manage and reduce treatment expenses:

1. Medication Cost Management

- **Prescription Assistance Programs**: Check if the manufacturer of your medication offers a patient assistance program. These programs can provide discounts or free medication to eligible patients.
- **Nonprofit Assistance**: Organizations such as the Partnership for Prescription Assistance (PPA) or the PAN Foundation offer support for people who struggle to pay for medications.
- **Pharmacy Savings Programs**: Enroll in pharmacy savings programs that can offer discounts on medications, even with insurance. Some large retailers and chain pharmacies provide these programs at no additional cost.

2. Reducing Doctor Visit Costs

- **Telemedicine Services**: Use telemedicine appointments for routine check-ups or prescription refills. These visits are often more affordable than in-person consultations.
- **Community Health Clinics**: Seek care from community health clinics that offer sliding-scale fees based on income. These clinics may provide reduced-cost care for patients without adequate insurance coverage.

3. Lab Tests and Diagnostic Procedures

- **Shop Around**: Prices for lab tests and diagnostic procedures can vary widely between facilities. Call different labs or use online price comparison tools to find the most affordable option.
- **Use In-Network Labs**: Ensure that the lab or facility is within your insurance network to minimize costs.

4. Emergency and Hospital Costs

- **Emergency Room Alternatives**: For non-life-threatening issues that need prompt attention, consider visiting urgent care centers instead of emergency rooms. Urgent care visits are typically much less expensive than emergency room visits.
- **Negotiate Medical Bills**: If you receive a large bill, contact the billing department to negotiate a payment plan or ask for a discount, especially if you can pay a lump sum.

10.4 Financial Assistance Options

When insurance and personal finances fall short, additional resources can help manage the costs of DI treatment:

1. Government Assistance Programs

- **Medicaid and State Health Programs**: If you meet income requirements, Medicaid or state health programs can help cover medical expenses, including medications and specialist visits.
- **Supplemental Security Income (SSI)**: Individuals with severe cases of DI that impact their ability to work may qualify for SSI, which provides financial assistance to cover living and medical costs.

2. Nonprofit and Charity Organizations

- **Patient Advocacy Groups**: Organizations such as the National Organization for Rare Disorders (NORD) offer grants and financial assistance for individuals with rare conditions, including DI.
- **Religious and Community Organizations**: Local charities or religious institutions may offer financial assistance for medical bills and related expenses.

3. Crowdfunding and Community Support

- **Crowdfunding Platforms**: Use platforms like GoFundMe to raise funds for medical expenses. Share your story with friends, family, and your community to gather support.
- **Local Fundraisers**: Organize or participate in local fundraising events that can help offset the costs of treatment and care.

4. Prescription Discount Programs

- **Discount Cards and Apps**: Programs like GoodRx, SingleCare, and Blink Health offer free or low-cost discount cards that can significantly reduce the cost of prescription medications.
- **Online Pharmacies**: Some licensed online pharmacies offer competitive pricing on prescription medications. Ensure the pharmacy is reputable and accredited.

10.5 Budgeting for DI Management

Creating and sticking to a budget is essential for managing the recurring expenses associated with DI:

1. Calculate Monthly Medical Expenses

- **Track Spending**: List all DI-related costs, including medications, doctor visits, lab tests, and health insurance premiums, to understand your monthly expenses.
- **Adjust as Needed**: Review your budget periodically and make adjustments based on changes in your treatment plan or medication costs.

2. Plan for Unexpected Costs

- **Emergency Fund**: Set aside a small amount each month into an emergency fund to cover unexpected medical expenses, such as ER visits or urgent care appointments.
- **Automatic Savings**: Set up an automatic transfer to a savings account specifically for medical expenses to ensure you're prepared for unforeseen costs.

3. Take Advantage of Tax Deductions

- **Medical Expense Deductions**: Keep track of your annual medical expenses. If they exceed 7.5% of your adjusted gross income (AGI), you may qualify for a tax deduction on your federal income taxes.
- **Save Receipts**: Maintain records of all medical expenses, including receipts and invoices, for tax purposes and potential reimbursement claims.

10.6 Navigating Financial Discussions with Healthcare Providers

Don't hesitate to discuss financial concerns with your healthcare providers. Here's how to approach these conversations:

1. Be Honest About Your Budget

- **Explain Your Situation**: Let your doctor know if you're having trouble affording your treatment plan. They may be able to suggest alternative medications, treatment plans, or provide samples to help reduce costs.
- **Ask About Cost-Effective Options**: Inquire if there are equally effective, lower-cost alternatives to your current medications or if extended-release options can reduce the frequency of doses.

2. Utilize Social Workers and Patient Advocates

- **Connect with a Social Worker**: Many hospitals and clinics have social workers or patient advocates who can help you navigate insurance issues and find financial assistance programs.

- **Patient Assistance Programs**: These advocates can assist with applications for patient assistance programs provided by drug manufacturers or nonprofit organizations.

Navigating the financial aspects of managing Diabetes Insipidus can be complex, but with the right knowledge and preparation, you can reduce stress and manage treatment costs more effectively. By leveraging insurance benefits, exploring financial assistance programs, and practicing smart cost management, you can focus on what matters most—maintaining your health and well-being.

Chapter 11: DI and the Mind – Mental Health and Resilience

Living with Diabetes Insipidus (DI) involves more than just physical management—it can also take a toll on mental health. The condition's symptoms, such as frequent urination, constant thirst, and the need for meticulous hydration management, can lead to stress, anxiety, and lifestyle disruptions. This chapter delves into coping with anxiety, managing lifestyle adjustments, and building resilience through support and mental health strategies.

11.1 The Mental Health Impact of DI

Understanding how DI affects mental health is the first step in building resilience. The daily challenges of managing DI can contribute to various emotional responses and psychological concerns, including:

1. Anxiety and Stress

- **Fear of Dehydration**: The constant need to stay hydrated and avoid dehydration can lead to chronic stress. Worrying about water access or managing sudden symptoms can increase anxiety, especially in social or unfamiliar settings.
- **Medical Anxiety**: Regular medical appointments, tests, and the need for ongoing medication can create feelings of anxiety and overwhelm.

2. Fatigue and Its Psychological Effects

- **Sleep Disruptions**: Nocturia (frequent nighttime urination) can interfere with sleep, leading to fatigue and its associated emotional impacts, such as irritability, reduced concentration, and mood swings.
- **Chronic Fatigue**: Persistent fatigue from disrupted sleep can contribute to feelings of helplessness and decreased motivation, affecting overall mental well-being.

3. Social Isolation and Embarrassment

- **Social Withdrawal**: Individuals with DI may avoid social activities due to the need for frequent restroom breaks or the constant presence of a water bottle. This can lead to feelings of isolation and loneliness.
- **Embarrassment**: The need for special accommodations or explaining the condition to others can cause embarrassment and self-consciousness, impacting self-esteem.

11.2 Coping Strategies for Anxiety and Stress

Managing anxiety and stress effectively is essential for maintaining mental well-being while living with DI. Here are practical strategies to help cope with these challenges:

1. Develop a Routine

- **Structured Daily Schedule**: Having a structured routine can help reduce the unpredictability that contributes to anxiety. Plan your day to include regular hydration times, breaks, and activities that align with your energy levels.
- **Preparation for Outings**: Plan ahead for activities that may require extra hydration or restroom access. Knowing that you have prepared for potential challenges can alleviate stress and boost confidence.

2. Practice Mindfulness and Relaxation Techniques

- **Deep Breathing Exercises**: Practicing deep breathing for a few minutes can help reduce acute stress and promote relaxation. Techniques such as the 4-7-8 breathing method (inhale for 4 seconds, hold for 7 seconds, exhale for 8 seconds) can be effective.

- **Guided Meditation**: Apps like Headspace, Calm, or Insight Timer offer guided meditations that can help you relax and refocus during stressful moments.
- **Progressive Muscle Relaxation (PMR)**: Tense and then relax different muscle groups, starting from your toes and working up to your head. This helps reduce physical tension and anxiety.

3. Cognitive Behavioral Techniques

- **Challenge Negative Thoughts**: When anxiety about your condition arises, practice challenging and reframing negative thoughts. For example, replace "I can't handle this" with "I've managed this before, and I have the tools to handle it again."
- **Journal Your Thoughts**: Keeping a journal can help you identify triggers and patterns in your thoughts and emotions, making it easier to develop coping strategies.

4. Limit Stress Triggers

- **Set Boundaries**: Limit exposure to stressors where possible, whether that means saying no to certain activities or taking on less responsibility when feeling overwhelmed.
- **Avoid Information Overload**: While it's important to be informed about your condition, avoid excessive research that may increase anxiety. Stick to reputable sources and consult with your healthcare provider for questions or concerns.

11.3 Adjusting Your Lifestyle to Support Mental Health

Adapting your lifestyle can help create a supportive environment that mitigates stress and enhances mental well-being:

1. Prioritize Sleep Hygiene

- **Create a Sleep-Conducive Environment**: Use blackout curtains, maintain a cool room temperature, and eliminate noise to improve sleep quality despite potential interruptions.
- **Limit Fluid Intake Before Bed**: Reduce water consumption a couple of hours before bedtime to minimize nighttime bathroom visits.
- **Relaxation Rituals**: Implement a pre-bedtime routine, such as reading or taking a warm bath, to signal your body that it's time to wind down.

2. Engage in Physical Activity

- **Exercise for Mental Clarity**: Regular physical activity, such as walking, yoga, or light strength training, can help reduce stress and anxiety by releasing endorphins.
- **Start Small**: If fatigue is an issue, start with short, low-intensity workouts and gradually build up as you feel more comfortable.

3. Create a Supportive Routine

- **Plan for Breaks**: Build breaks into your daily schedule to rest and reset. This can help prevent burnout and maintain energy throughout the day.
- **Hydration-Friendly Meals**: Incorporate meals that support hydration without contributing to increased thirst. Foods high in water content, such as fruits and vegetables, can help maintain balance.

11.4 Seeking Support and Building Resilience

Connecting with others and building a network of support is vital for long-term resilience and mental health.

1. Reach Out to Friends and Family

- **Communicate Your Needs**: Let friends and family know how they can support you, whether it's by understanding your need for frequent breaks or helping you prepare for an outing.
- **Stay Connected**: Make an effort to maintain social connections, even if it's through virtual hangouts or phone calls. Social interaction can help prevent isolation and boost mood.

2. Join Support Groups

- **Online Communities**: Participating in online support groups for DI or chronic health conditions can provide a sense of community and shared understanding. Platforms like Facebook and specific health-focused forums can be great places to connect.
- **Local Support Groups**: If available, join local groups for chronic illness support to meet people face-to-face who understand the challenges you face.

3. Professional Mental Health Support

- **Therapists and Counselors**: Consider seeing a therapist or counselor, particularly one experienced with chronic illness or health-related anxiety. Cognitive Behavioral Therapy (CBT) and other therapeutic approaches can be highly effective in managing anxiety and stress.
- **Psychiatric Consultation**: If anxiety or depression becomes severe, a psychiatrist may be able to provide medical treatment or medication to support your mental health alongside therapy.

11.5 Building Long-Term Resilience

Resilience is the ability to bounce back from challenges, adapt, and thrive despite adversity. Here's how to build resilience while living with DI:

1. Focus on Strengths and Achievements

- **Celebrate Small Wins**: Recognize and celebrate your accomplishments, whether it's successfully managing your symptoms during a busy day or learning new coping skills.
- **Set Realistic Goals**: Set achievable short- and long-term goals to maintain motivation and a sense of purpose.

2. Maintain a Positive Outlook

- **Practice Gratitude**: Regularly acknowledging things you are grateful for can shift your focus away from challenges and toward positive aspects of life. Keep a gratitude journal to jot down daily reflections.
- **Emphasize Growth**: View setbacks as opportunities for learning and growth rather than as failures.

3. Develop Problem-Solving Skills

- **Anticipate Challenges**: Think ahead about potential problems and create action plans for how you will address them.
- **Be Adaptable**: Flexibility is key when living with a chronic condition. Be open to changing your strategies and routines as needed to maintain well-being.

4. Practice Self-Compassion

- **Be Kind to Yourself**: Treat yourself with the same kindness and understanding that you would offer to a friend. Remember that it's okay to have difficult days, and not every day will go as planned.

- **Avoid Comparison**: Resist comparing your experiences with others, even those with the same condition. Each person's journey is unique, and progress may look different from one person to another.

Building resilience and managing mental health effectively while living with Diabetes Insipidus requires a combination of self-awareness, strategic coping mechanisms, and a supportive network. By implementing the tips and strategies in this chapter, you can develop a balanced approach that nurtures your mental well-being and empowers you to face life's challenges with confidence.

Chapter 12: Restful Nights – Managing DI and Sleep Quality

For individuals with Diabetes Insipidus (DI), achieving a restful night's sleep can be particularly challenging due to the condition's hallmark symptom: frequent urination, including at night (nocturia). Poor sleep quality can lead to fatigue, decreased concentration, irritability, and overall diminished quality of life. This chapter focuses on strategies to manage nighttime symptoms, maintain sleep hygiene, and utilize sleep aids to improve sleep quality while living with DI.

12.1 Understanding Nocturia and Its Impact

Nocturia, the need to wake up multiple times during the night to urinate, is a common issue for those with DI. This disruption can affect the sleep cycle and lead to fragmented sleep, making it difficult to achieve the restorative rest needed for optimal health.

Why Nocturia Occurs in DI:

- **Impaired Water Retention**: Due to insufficient or ineffective antidiuretic hormone (ADH) activity, the kidneys produce large amounts of dilute urine. This continues during the night, leading to the frequent need to urinate.
- **Increased Thirst**: Excessive thirst (polydipsia) can also contribute to nighttime water consumption, exacerbating nocturia.

Consequences of Frequent Nighttime Urination:

- **Interrupted Sleep Cycle**: Frequent awakenings disrupt the sleep cycle, particularly deep sleep stages, which are essential for physical and mental recovery.
- **Fatigue and Daytime Sleepiness**: Chronic sleep interruptions can lead to daytime drowsiness, reduced cognitive function, and lower productivity.
- **Mood Changes**: Poor sleep quality can increase irritability, anxiety, and even depression over time.

12.2 Strategies to Manage Nocturia

While it may not be possible to eliminate nocturia entirely, there are strategies that can help reduce its frequency and impact on sleep quality:

1. Timing Fluid Intake

- **Limit Fluids Before Bed**: Reduce fluid intake 1-2 hours before bedtime to help decrease urine production during the night. Ensure you meet your hydration needs earlier in the day.
- **Pre-Bed Hydration**: If you need to drink water before bed, take small sips rather than large amounts to avoid stimulating urine production.

2. Adjust Medication Timing

- **Evening Medication Adjustments**: Work with your healthcare provider to adjust the timing of medications like desmopressin to align with your sleep schedule. Taking a dose in the evening may help reduce urine output during the night.
- **Avoid Diuretics Late in the Day**: If you take diuretics as part of your DI treatment plan, ensure they are taken earlier in the day to minimize nighttime effects.

3. Optimize Bathroom Access

- **Strategic Placement**: Position your bed closer to the bathroom if possible to reduce the time it takes to get up and return to bed, minimizing sleep disruption.
- **Night Lights**: Use low-intensity night lights in the hallway and bathroom to avoid fully waking yourself with bright lights during trips to the restroom.

12.3 Maintaining Sleep Hygiene

Good sleep hygiene practices can help improve the overall quality of sleep, even when nocturia is present:

1. Create a Sleep-Friendly Environment

- **Comfortable Bed**: Invest in a supportive mattress and pillows that promote comfort and help you fall back asleep quickly after being awakened.
- **Dark and Quiet Room**: Use blackout curtains or an eye mask to block out light and earplugs or a white noise machine to mask disruptive sounds.
- **Cool Temperature**: Maintain a slightly cooler room temperature (around 60-67°F or 15-19°C), as this can promote deeper sleep.

2. Establish a Consistent Sleep Schedule

- **Regular Sleep-Wake Times**: Go to bed and wake up at the same time each day, even on weekends, to regulate your body's internal clock.
- **Wind-Down Routine**: Create a relaxing pre-sleep routine, such as reading, gentle stretching, or practicing mindfulness, to signal your body that it's time to sleep.

3. Limit Stimulants

- **Avoid Caffeine**: Refrain from consuming caffeine in the afternoon and evening, as it can interfere with falling asleep.
- **Reduce Screen Time**: Minimize exposure to screens (phones, tablets, computers) at least an hour before bedtime. The blue

light emitted by screens can suppress melatonin production and delay sleep onset.

12.4 Sleep Aids and Interventions

For those who continue to struggle with sleep despite implementing lifestyle changes, additional sleep aids and interventions may be beneficial:

1. Over-the-Counter Sleep Aids

- **Melatonin Supplements**: Melatonin is a hormone that helps regulate sleep. Taking melatonin supplements before bed may help you fall asleep faster and improve sleep quality.
- **Herbal Remedies**: Natural sleep aids such as valerian root, chamomile tea, or magnesium supplements can promote relaxation and support better sleep.

2. Prescription Sleep Medications

- **Consult with a Doctor**: If over-the-counter options do not help, speak with your doctor about prescription sleep aids. These medications should be used cautiously and typically only for short-term support due to potential side effects and the risk of dependency.

3. Cognitive Behavioral Therapy for Insomnia (CBT-I)

- **Structured Sleep Therapy**: CBT-I is an evidence-based treatment that helps address the thoughts and behaviors contributing to poor sleep. It can be highly effective for individuals with chronic insomnia related to medical conditions like DI.
- **Guided Sessions**: CBT-I can be conducted with a trained therapist or through online programs and apps designed for sleep improvement.

12.5 Managing Disruptions and Returning to Sleep

Even with the best preparation, nighttime awakenings may still occur. Knowing how to handle these interruptions can help you fall back asleep more easily:

1. Practice Relaxation Techniques

- **Deep Breathing**: Use deep breathing exercises, such as diaphragmatic breathing, to calm your nervous system and prepare your body to return to sleep.
- **Progressive Relaxation**: Tense and release different muscle groups while lying in bed to release physical tension and promote relaxation.

2. Avoid Checking the Clock

- **Turn Your Clock Away**: Watching the clock can increase anxiety about not sleeping and make it harder to drift off again. Turn your clock away from your line of sight to reduce stress.

3. Get Out of Bed if Necessary

- **Briefly Leave the Bedroom**: If you find yourself lying awake for more than 20 minutes, get out of bed and do a quiet, non-stimulating activity like reading or listening to calming music until you feel sleepy again.
- **Keep the Lights Low**: Use minimal lighting to avoid fully waking your body's alertness system.

12.6 Long-Term Strategies for Improved Sleep Quality

Achieving consistent, high-quality sleep may take time and require the integration of multiple strategies:

1. Monitor Your Sleep Patterns

- **Sleep Diary**: Keep a journal to track your sleep patterns, nighttime awakenings, and related factors like fluid intake and medication timing. This can help identify trends and areas for improvement.
- **Sleep Apps**: Consider using a sleep-tracking app that provides data on sleep duration, quality, and disturbances to better understand how DI affects your sleep.

2. Collaborate with Your Healthcare Provider

- **Discuss Adjustments**: Work with your doctor to adjust medication doses or try new treatments that might reduce nighttime urination.
- **Regular Check-Ups**: Regular medical check-ups can help monitor your overall health and address any new or worsening symptoms that impact sleep.

3. Stay Consistent

- **Stick to Your Routine**: Consistency is key when it comes to sleep hygiene and managing nocturia. Sticking to your sleep schedule and pre-bed routine can help reinforce healthy sleep habits over time.

12.7 Supporting Overall Health to Improve Sleep

Beyond DI-specific strategies, overall health and wellness practices can contribute to better sleep:

1. Maintain a Balanced Diet

- **Hydration-Friendly Foods**: Include foods that support hydration and avoid excessive salt intake, which can increase thirst.
- **Nutrient-Rich Meals**: Ensure your diet includes nutrients like magnesium and potassium, which support muscle relaxation and sleep quality.

2. Regular Physical Activity

- **Daytime Exercise**: Engage in moderate physical activity during the day, as this can promote better sleep quality. Avoid vigorous exercise close to bedtime, as it may increase alertness.
- **Light Evening Activities**: If needed, light stretching or yoga in the evening can help your body unwind before bed.

3. Manage Stress

- **Daily Relaxation Practices**: Incorporate stress-reducing activities such as journaling, meditation, or spending time outdoors to support overall mental health and better sleep.
- **Mindfulness Practices**: Mindfulness techniques can help reduce anxiety, making it easier to fall asleep and stay asleep throughout the night.

Achieving restful nights with DI may require a combination of strategies, from managing fluid intake and optimizing medication timing to maintaining good sleep hygiene and exploring sleep aids. By implementing the advice in this chapter, individuals with DI can improve their sleep quality, support overall well-being, and enhance their ability to manage daily life effectively.

Chapter 13: Supporting Young Ones – DI in Children

Managing Diabetes Insipidus (DI) in children presents unique challenges that can impact their physical health, emotional well-being, and overall development. Parents, caregivers, and educators play a crucial role in creating an environment that supports the child's growth while addressing the symptoms and complications of DI. This chapter provides an in-depth look at managing DI in young children, understanding the distinct challenges they face, and strategies to support their growth and well-being.

13.1 Understanding the Unique Challenges of DI in Children

DI can affect children differently than adults due to their developing bodies and the demands of growth. Recognizing these challenges is essential for providing effective support.

1. Rapid Dehydration

- **Increased Risk**: Children are more vulnerable to dehydration because they have a higher body water content than adults and may not recognize or express the need for water adequately.
- **Frequent Urination**: Constant trips to the bathroom can disrupt daily activities, including school and playtime, making it difficult for children to fully engage in normal childhood experiences.

2. Communication Barriers

- **Limited Vocabulary**: Younger children may have difficulty communicating their symptoms, such as thirst or the urgency to urinate.
- **Unfamiliarity with Symptoms**: A child with newly diagnosed DI may not understand what is happening to their body or how to articulate their needs.

3. Emotional and Social Implications

- **Peer Interactions**: Children with DI may feel different from their peers due to frequent water intake, restroom breaks, or medical routines. This can lead to feelings of embarrassment or isolation.
- **Self-Esteem**: Repeated disruptions in school or social activities can impact a child's self-confidence and make them more self-conscious.

13.2 Managing DI in Children: Day-to-Day Strategies

Creating a structured and supportive daily routine can help manage DI symptoms effectively while allowing children to participate in activities and thrive.

1. Hydration Management

- **Scheduled Hydration**: Establish regular times throughout the day for the child to drink water. This helps maintain hydration without overwhelming their bladder.
- **Portable Water Solutions**: Provide the child with a fun, kid-friendly water bottle that they can take to school or on outings to encourage drinking water regularly.
- **Electrolyte Balance**: Supplement hydration with electrolyte solutions to ensure that essential minerals like sodium and potassium are replenished.

2. Bathroom Access

- **Frequent Breaks**: Ensure the child has easy and unrestricted access to restrooms, both at home and in school. Communicate with teachers and school staff to establish a plan that allows the child to use the restroom whenever necessary without needing permission.
- **Overnight Management**: For children who experience nocturia, consider strategies like limiting fluid intake an hour or two before bedtime and using absorbent bed pads to manage nighttime accidents.

3. Medication Adherence

- **Consistent Routine**: Administer medications like desmopressin at the same times each day to create a predictable schedule that the child can adapt to.
- **Child-Friendly Formats**: If available, choose medication formats that are easier for children to take, such as flavored dissolvable tablets or liquid forms.

13.3 Supporting Emotional and Social Development

Managing DI in children is not just about physical health; it also involves fostering emotional resilience and social integration.

1. Encourage Open Communication

- **Teach Children to Express Their Needs**: Help children develop the language they need to communicate symptoms like thirst, urgency, or discomfort. Simple phrases like "I need a drink of water" or "I need to use the restroom" can be reinforced at home and at school.
- **Active Listening**: Listen to the child's concerns and feelings about living with DI. Validate their experiences and reassure them that it's okay to ask for help or feel different at times.

2. Build Confidence

- **Celebrate Small Wins**: Recognize and celebrate when the child manages their DI well, such as remembering to drink water on their own or taking their medication without prompting.
- **Support Social Activities**: Encourage participation in activities and playdates with friends. Make necessary accommodations, such as bringing extra water or planning bathroom breaks, to ensure they can join in comfortably.

3. Address Peer Awareness

- **Educate Peers**: In school settings, consider discussing DI in an age-appropriate way with the child's classmates to promote understanding and prevent teasing. Ensure this is done with the child's consent and in a way that makes them feel comfortable.

- **Normalize the Condition**: Emphasize that many people have unique health needs and that managing DI is just one way of taking care of oneself.

13.4 Creating a Supportive Environment at School

A well-coordinated approach between parents, teachers, and school administrators can create a supportive learning environment for a child with DI.

1. Develop a School Plan

- **504 Plan or IEP**: Work with the school to create a 504 Plan or Individualized Education Program (IEP) that outlines accommodations such as unlimited restroom access, permission to carry a water bottle, and allowances for extra snacks if needed.
- **Teacher Communication**: Keep teachers informed about the child's condition and provide them with information on how to support the child during school hours.

2. Manage Extracurricular Activities

- **Discuss Needs with Coaches**: If the child participates in sports or after-school activities, inform coaches or group leaders about DI and any accommodations that may be necessary, such as additional water breaks.
- **Field Trips**: Coordinate with teachers to ensure field trips are planned with restroom and water access in mind. Provide a kit with water, medication, and a note explaining the child's condition for caregivers or teachers on the trip.

13.5 Tips for Parents and Caregivers

Parents and caregivers play a vital role in managing DI for young children. Here are additional tips to support both the child's health and emotional well-being:

1. Foster Independence

- **Teach Self-Management Skills**: As children grow, encourage them to take on age-appropriate responsibilities, such as carrying their water bottle, taking their medication, and recognizing when they need a restroom break.
- **Involve Them in Their Care**: Let children be part of their care routine by allowing them to choose their water bottles, set hydration reminders, or help prepare their medication. This fosters a sense of control and responsibility.

2. Stay Organized

- **Keep a Medical Journal**: Track symptoms, water intake, and medication times to spot any patterns or issues that may need adjusting.
- **Plan for Emergencies**: Pack an emergency kit that includes water, medication, a change of clothes, and a medical ID card. This can be taken on family outings or to school for peace of mind.

3. Prioritize Self-Care for Caregivers

- **Manage Caregiver Stress**: Caring for a child with DI can be demanding. Take time for your own self-care to avoid burnout and maintain the energy needed to support your child.
- **Seek Support**: Join support groups or online forums where parents of children with DI share experiences and advice. Connect-

ing with others in similar situations can provide reassurance and helpful tips.

13.6 Monitoring Growth and Development

Children with DI need regular monitoring to ensure they are growing and developing appropriately, as chronic dehydration and electrolyte imbalances can impact growth.

1. Regular Check-Ups

- **Routine Pediatric Appointments**: Schedule regular check-ups with a pediatrician and, if necessary, a pediatric endocrinologist. These specialists can monitor the child's growth, weight, and hydration status and adjust treatment as needed.
- **Blood Tests**: Periodic blood tests may be recommended to monitor electrolyte levels and ensure there are no deficiencies or imbalances.

2. Nutritional Support

- **Balanced Diet**: Ensure the child receives a diet rich in essential nutrients, including calcium, magnesium, and potassium, to support growth and development.
- **Hydration-Focused Foods**: Include water-rich foods like fruits and vegetables in their diet to help maintain hydration levels naturally.

3. Growth Milestones

- **Track Growth Progress**: Keep a record of the child's height and weight milestones. Significant deviations from expected growth patterns should be discussed with a healthcare provider.
- **Address Concerns Early**: If you notice any signs of stunted growth, persistent fatigue, or developmental delays, consult a

doctor for a comprehensive evaluation and potential treatment adjustments.

13.7 Building Long-Term Resilience

Helping children develop resilience is essential for them to navigate the challenges of DI as they grow.

1. Teach Problem-Solving Skills

- **Encourage Self-Advocacy**: Teach children to express their needs clearly and advocate for themselves in different environments, such as asking for a water refill at school or reminding a teacher about a restroom break.
- **Role-Playing Scenarios**: Practice different situations where the child might need to explain their condition or request support. This helps build confidence and preparedness.

2. Cultivate a Positive Mindset

- **Focus on Strengths**: Emphasize the child's strengths and achievements outside of their condition, reinforcing the idea that DI is just one aspect of who they are.
- **Model Resilience**: Show how you cope with challenges as a caregiver, providing a positive example for the child to follow.

3. Encourage Open Dialogue

- **Create a Safe Space**: Make sure the child feels comfortable discussing their feelings about DI. Let them know it's okay to express frustration, sadness, or worry and that you're there to listen and support them.
- **Regular Check-Ins**: Have regular conversations to see how they're coping emotionally and socially. This helps identify any

issues early and provides an opportunity for reassurance and support.

Managing DI in children requires a holistic approach that includes physical care, emotional support, and proactive planning. By implementing the strategies outlined in this chapter, parents, caregivers, and educators can help children with DI lead full, active lives while building the resilience they need to navigate future challenges with confidence.

Chapter 14: Building Community – Advocacy and Support Networks

Living with Diabetes Insipidus (DI) can be an isolating experience, especially when those around you may not understand the condition. However, connecting with a community, finding support, and advocating for awareness can make a significant difference in how individuals and families navigate life with DI. This chapter will guide you through the importance of joining DI communities, finding reliable support networks, and participating in advocacy efforts to spread awareness and support others with the condition.

14.1 The Importance of Community in Managing DI

Being part of a community can provide a sense of belonging and reduce feelings of isolation. Connecting with others who share similar experiences can offer emotional support, practical advice, and new perspectives on managing DI effectively.

1. Emotional Support

- **Shared Experiences**: Engaging with others who understand the challenges of DI can create a sense of camaraderie and validation. It's reassuring to know that you are not alone and that others have faced similar obstacles.
- **Peer Encouragement**: Fellow community members can offer encouragement and support during tough times, whether you're dealing with new symptoms, treatment adjustments, or lifestyle changes.

2. Knowledge Sharing

- **Exchange of Ideas**: Communities often share strategies for managing DI that you may not have considered, such as tips for staying hydrated, managing medications, or navigating social situations.

- **Learning from Others**: Hearing about other people's experiences can provide insights into different treatments, products, or techniques that may be beneficial.

3. Advocacy and Awareness

- **Raising Awareness**: Joining an advocacy group or support network gives you the chance to spread awareness about DI and educate others, fostering greater understanding and empathy.
- **Driving Change**: Advocacy can lead to improvements in policies, research funding, and healthcare practices that benefit everyone affected by DI.

14.2 Finding and Joining DI Support Networks

Finding the right support network can make a significant impact on your journey with DI. Here's how to locate and join these communities:

1. Online Communities

- **Social Media Groups**: Platforms such as Facebook have groups dedicated to chronic health conditions, including DI. These groups allow for real-time discussions, sharing resources, and building connections.
- **Forums and Health Websites**: Websites like Reddit and specialized health forums have sections where people discuss DI, share their experiences, and offer support.
- **Condition-Specific Platforms**: Some websites and organizations are designed specifically for DI or rare conditions, providing forums, educational resources, and a space for connecting with others.

2. Local Support Groups

- **Community Centers and Hospitals**: Check local community centers or hospitals for support groups that focus on chronic conditions. While DI-specific groups may be rare, groups for general rare diseases or chronic illness management can also be beneficial.
- **Specialty Clinics**: Endocrinology clinics may have information on support groups or may host their own sessions where patients can connect.

3. Nonprofit Organizations and Advocacy Groups

- **National and International Organizations**: Groups such as the National Organization for Rare Disorders (NORD) and the Rare Disease United Foundation often have resources or can connect you to DI-specific support.
- **Health Foundations**: Reach out to foundations that support endocrine or kidney health. They may offer educational webinars, conferences, or local meet-ups.
- **Webinars and Online Conferences**: Participating in online events hosted by these organizations can expand your knowledge and connect you with experts and peers.

14.3 Building Your Personal Support Network

A strong personal support network made up of family, friends, and close acquaintances is equally important for managing DI effectively.

1. Educating Your Inner Circle

- **Informative Conversations**: Take the time to explain what DI is, how it affects you, and what kind of support you may need from your loved ones. Use simple terms to help them understand your condition without overwhelming details.
- **Resource Sharing**: Provide family and friends with resources, such as educational pamphlets, reputable websites, or videos that explain DI. This helps them learn more at their own pace.

2. Encouraging Empathy and Understanding

- **Explain Your Symptoms**: Help your support network understand common symptoms, like excessive thirst, frequent urination, and potential fatigue. This prepares them to be patient and supportive when symptoms arise.
- **Address Misconceptions**: Clarify any misconceptions about DI, such as confusing it with diabetes mellitus. Explaining the differences can foster better understanding and reduce frustration or misunderstandings.

3. Involving Your Support Network in Care

- **Shared Responsibilities**: If you need help managing your symptoms or treatment, involve trusted individuals in your care. This could include helping with medication schedules, driving to appointments, or simply being there to offer emotional support.
- **Backup Plans**: Create a plan that outlines what friends or family should do in case of an emergency, such as sudden dehydration or a medical issue. This gives everyone involved peace of mind and a clear course of action.

14.4 Spreading Awareness and Advocacy

Advocating for DI awareness benefits not only individuals directly affected but also promotes understanding within the broader community.

1. Participating in Awareness Campaigns

- **Join Existing Campaigns**: Participate in awareness initiatives organized by DI-focused nonprofits or rare disease advocacy groups. Share their posts on social media, attend their events, and contribute where you can.
- **Create Your Own Awareness Efforts**: Use platforms like social media or local community events to spread awareness about DI. You can write blog posts, create videos, or host Q&A sessions to educate others.

2. Sharing Your Story

- **Personal Testimonies**: Sharing your personal journey with DI can be a powerful way to raise awareness and inspire others. Consider writing an article, participating in interviews, or speaking at health-related events.
- **Social Media Platforms**: Use social media to share your experiences, post tips for managing DI, or connect with others. Hashtags like #DiabetesInsipidus, #RareDiseaseAwareness, or #LivingWithDI can help your story reach more people.

3. Supporting Policy Changes

- **Advocate for Healthcare Policy**: Join efforts that push for better healthcare policies that impact rare disease management, such as improved access to medications, more comprehensive insurance coverage, or increased research funding.

- **Contact Legislators**: Reach out to local or national legislators to share your story and advocate for changes that could improve the lives of those with DI and other rare conditions.

14.5 Involving Children and Teens with DI in Community Building

If your child has DI, involving them in community-building efforts can help them feel less alone and more empowered.

1. Age-Appropriate Involvement

- **Youth-Friendly Communities**: Find or create DI groups that are tailored to children or teenagers. These groups can include activities, mentorship programs, and fun ways for young people to connect.
- **Encourage Participation**: Allow children to take part in community events, whether online or in-person, so they can meet others their age with similar experiences.

2. Family Engagement

- **Family Support Groups**: Join family-based support groups that address DI management collectively. This provides both the child and parents with a network of understanding peers and caregivers.
- **Educational Workshops**: Attend workshops designed for children and families to learn about DI in an engaging and interactive manner. These events often offer practical tips and foster a sense of community.

3. Teaching Self-Advocacy

- **Empower Young Voices**: Encourage older children and teens to speak about their experiences, whether through school presentations, social media, or involvement in awareness campaigns.
- **Teach Communication Skills**: Help children develop the language and confidence to explain DI to their friends, teachers, or classmates. This not only fosters understanding but also empowers them to advocate for themselves.

14.6 Tips for Sustaining Engagement in DI Communities
Staying active in DI communities and advocacy efforts can provide long-term benefits. Here are some tips for sustaining engagement:
1. Balance Participation

- **Avoid Burnout**: Be mindful of your energy levels and commitments to avoid feeling overwhelmed. It's okay to take breaks from advocacy or participation and return when you're ready.
- **Prioritize Self-Care**: Engage in activities that recharge you, whether they're related to DI or not. Maintaining a balanced life helps keep your advocacy efforts sustainable.

2. Connect with Key Members

- **Identify Mentors and Peers**: Build relationships with people in the community who inspire you or share similar experiences. They can provide mentorship, advice, and support.
- **Collaborate on Projects**: Work with others to create joint awareness campaigns, co-author blog posts, or organize community events. Collaboration can make advocacy more effective and fulfilling.

3. Stay Informed

- **Keep Learning**: Stay updated on new research, treatment options, and policy changes related to DI. This information can make your advocacy more impactful and keep you motivated to stay involved.
- **Attend Conferences**: If possible, attend rare disease or DI-specific conferences. These events are excellent opportunities to learn, meet others, and find inspiration for new advocacy projects.

Building a strong DI community and participating in advocacy can enhance your support network, raise awareness, and contribute to a greater sense of purpose and connection. Whether you're a person with DI, a caregiver, or a supporter, taking the time to engage with others and spread awareness helps build a more informed and compassionate world. By following the strategies outlined in this chapter, you can find or create the community support you need and contribute to a positive impact for all those affected by DI.

Chapter 15: Living Well Long-Term – Lifestyle Tips for Thriving with DI

Diabetes Insipidus (DI) requires continuous management and lifestyle adjustments to maintain overall health and well-being. Living with DI is more than just managing symptoms; it's about developing a sustainable lifestyle that allows you to thrive and adapt over time. This chapter offers comprehensive, practical tips for thriving with DI and adjusting routines to align with evolving needs and life stages.

15.1 Embracing a DI-Friendly Lifestyle

Understanding how to integrate DI management into your daily life is the foundation for long-term well-being. Embracing these habits can make living with DI more manageable and less disruptive.

1. Prioritize Hydration Consistently

- **Scheduled Hydration**: Establish a routine for drinking water throughout the day to prevent dehydration. Small, frequent sips are more effective than consuming large amounts all at once.
- **Keep Water Accessible**: Carry a water bottle at all times, whether you're at work, home, or out running errands. Choose bottles that are portable, insulated, and easy to refill.
- **Hydration Aids**: Incorporate electrolyte solutions or drinks that help maintain balance without overloading on plain water. This is particularly important during physical activity or hot weather.

2. Optimize Diet for Hydration and Health

- **Water-Rich Foods**: Include foods like cucumbers, watermelon, oranges, and leafy greens in your diet to supplement hydration naturally.
- **Balanced Nutrition**: Maintain a diet rich in nutrients that support energy levels and overall health. Focus on lean proteins, whole grains, healthy fats, and a variety of vegetables and fruits.
- **Limit High-Sodium Foods**: Excessive salt intake can increase thirst and potentially lead to dehydration. Monitor your salt consumption and choose low-sodium options when possible.

3. Monitor Symptoms Regularly

- **Daily Tracking**: Keep a journal or use a mobile app to track water intake, urination frequency, and other symptoms. This can help you notice trends and adjust your habits as needed.
- **Body Cues**: Learn to recognize early signs of dehydration (such as dry mouth, dizziness, or dark urine) and take proactive measures to rehydrate.

15.2 Developing Adaptive Routines

Adapting your daily routines over time helps integrate DI management seamlessly into your lifestyle.

1. Morning Routine

- **Start with Hydration**: Begin your day with a glass of water to replenish fluids lost overnight.
- **Medication Management**: Take any prescribed medications, such as desmopressin, at a consistent time each morning. Set reminders if needed to ensure adherence.
- **Plan Your Day**: Outline your daily activities and identify when and where you'll have access to water and restrooms.

2. Work or School Routine

- **Hydration Strategy**: Set up a system for regular water breaks. If possible, establish a routine that aligns with your workload, class schedule, or daily meetings.
- **Restroom Planning**: Choose a workstation or seat in classrooms that allows easy access to restrooms. Notify teachers or supervisors about your needs discreetly to avoid disruption.
- **Pack Essentials**: Carry a hydration kit that includes a water bottle, electrolyte packets, and any necessary snacks that help maintain energy.

3. Evening Routine

- **Gradual Fluid Reduction**: Reduce water intake an hour or two before bedtime to minimize nocturnal urination, while still ensuring you're hydrated enough for restful sleep.
- **Reflect and Adjust**: Take a few moments to reflect on how your day went in terms of symptom management. Make notes on any adjustments needed for the next day.
- **Wind Down**: Engage in relaxing activities that help signal to your body that it's time for rest. This can include reading, stretching, or listening to calming music.

15.3 Staying Active and Healthy

Physical activity and wellness are essential for long-term health. Here's how to stay active while managing DI effectively:

1. Choose DI-Compatible Workouts

- **Low to Moderate Intensity**: Opt for activities that don't lead to excessive sweating and fluid loss, such as walking, swimming, or yoga.
- **Hydrate Before, During, and After**: Plan your hydration before starting any exercise, take sips of water throughout your workout, and replenish fluids afterward.
- **Monitor Your Body**: Pay attention to signs of overexertion or dehydration, such as lightheadedness or excessive fatigue. Adjust the intensity or duration as needed.

2. Incorporate Flexibility

- **Adapt Based on Weather**: During hot or humid days, shift workouts to cooler times, such as early morning or late evening. For cold days, ensure you stay hydrated even if you don't feel as thirsty.
- **Exercise Alternatives**: When outdoor conditions aren't ideal, consider indoor activities like at-home workouts or gym sessions.

3. Maintain an Active Lifestyle Beyond Workouts

- **Daily Movement**: Incorporate small, active habits into your day, like taking the stairs, stretching during breaks, or going for short walks.
- **Stay Socially Active**: Join activity groups or classes that align with your interests and encourage you to stay engaged and connected with others.

15.4 Managing Social and Recreational Activities

Socializing and recreational activities don't have to be limited by DI. Here are some tips for enjoying life while managing your condition:

1. Prepare for Social Gatherings

- **Communicate Your Needs**: Let close friends or hosts know in advance that you may need frequent restroom access or extra water. This helps avoid any awkwardness and ensures they're prepared to accommodate you.
- **Plan for Hydration**: Bring your own water bottle and electrolyte packets to events. Having your hydration supplies on hand can make social outings less stressful.

2. Eating Out

- **Choose Hydration-Friendly Meals**: Opt for dishes that aren't overly salty or spicy, as these can increase thirst. Meals with plenty of vegetables or water-rich sides are beneficial.
- **Order Smart**: Request water or a low-sugar electrolyte drink at restaurants and take small sips throughout the meal to stay hydrated.

3. Traveling with DI

- **Pack a Travel Kit**: Include water bottles, electrolytes, medication, and a small notebook with important health information and contact numbers.
- **Research Restroom Locations**: Know where restrooms are located at airports, train stations, and other travel hubs.

- **Plan Accommodations**: Stay in places that offer easy access to water and restrooms, such as hotels with in-room amenities like water dispensers or fridges.

15.5 Leveraging Technology for DI Management

Technology can streamline DI management and help you maintain consistency over time:

1. Hydration Apps

- **Tracking Fluid Intake**: Use hydration apps to monitor your daily water intake and set reminders to drink water at regular intervals.
- **Analyzing Trends**: Apps with trend analysis can help you identify patterns in your symptoms and make necessary adjustments to your hydration strategy.

2. Medication Reminders

- **Smart Reminders**: Use smartphone apps or wearables to remind you when it's time to take your medication.
- **Integrated Health Platforms**: Consider using health apps that allow you to track medication, hydration, and symptoms in one place for a comprehensive overview.

3. Online Support Groups

- **Connect Virtually**: Join online forums and support groups to exchange tips, share experiences, and gain motivation from others living with DI.
- **Educational Resources**: Stay informed about new treatment options or lifestyle tips by subscribing to newsletters or following reliable DI-focused health websites.

15.6 Adjusting Routines as Life Changes

Life changes, such as starting a new job, going to college, or entering different life stages, may require adjustments to how you manage DI:

1. Transitioning to New Environments

- **Plan Ahead**: When starting a new job or attending school, scout out water and restroom facilities in advance and discuss accommodations with your employer or school administration.
- **Create a Routine**: Establish a new daily routine that aligns with your new schedule, ensuring that it incorporates hydration, medication, and breaks.

2. Adapting During Major Life Changes

- **Pregnancy and DI**: Consult with your healthcare provider for personalized advice on managing DI during pregnancy, as hormone changes may impact symptoms and treatment needs.
- **Aging with DI**: As you age, your body's hydration needs and response to treatment may change. Regular check-ups with a healthcare provider can help adjust your management plan as necessary.

3. Preparing for Emergency Situations

- **Emergency Kit**: Keep an emergency kit that includes water, medication, and electrolyte solutions for unforeseen situations, such as natural disasters or power outages.
- **Medical ID**: Wear a medical alert bracelet or carry an ID card that provides information about your condition and emergency contacts.

15.7 Building a Positive Mindset for Long-Term Well-Being

Maintaining a positive mindset is crucial for thriving with DI over the long term:

1. Practice Gratitude

- **Daily Reflection**: Take a few minutes each day to reflect on what you're grateful for. This practice can shift your focus from challenges to the positive aspects of your life.
- **Acknowledge Progress**: Celebrate milestones and personal achievements, no matter how small. Recognize the effort you put into managing your health.

2. Embrace Flexibility

- **Adapt When Needed**: Life with DI may require changes to your routines or approaches. Embrace flexibility and be willing to try new strategies to maintain your well-being.
- **Learn from Setbacks**: When things don't go as planned, view setbacks as learning experiences and use them to refine your management plan.

3. Stay Connected

- **Maintain Social Connections**: Relationships can provide emotional support and motivation. Stay connected with friends, family, and community groups to foster a sense of belonging.
- **Involvement in DI Communities**: Engage in advocacy or support networks where you can share your experiences, learn from others, and contribute to awareness efforts.

Living well with Diabetes Insipidus involves a balance of proactive planning, adaptive routines, and a supportive mindset. By integrating these practical tips into your daily life and adjusting as needed, you can thrive while managing DI and enjoy a fulfilling, active lifestyle.

Appendices

Appendix A: Glossary of Terms

Understanding medical and condition-specific terminology is essential for managing Diabetes Insipidus (DI) effectively. This glossary provides detailed definitions of key terms used throughout this guide to help clarify medical concepts, treatment options, and lifestyle considerations.

1. Antidiuretic Hormone (ADH): Also known as vasopressin, this hormone is produced by the hypothalamus and stored in the pituitary gland. It helps the kidneys manage the amount of water in the body by reducing urine production. In DI, the body may have insufficient ADH or resistance to it, leading to excessive urination.

2. Central Diabetes Insipidus (CDI): A type of DI caused by damage to the hypothalamus or pituitary gland, which affects the production or release of ADH. This damage can be due to injury, surgery, tumors, or genetic disorders.

3. Nephrogenic Diabetes Insipidus (NDI): A form of DI where the kidneys do not respond properly to ADH, even though it is being produced normally. This can be caused by genetic factors, chronic kidney disease, or certain medications.

4. Gestational Diabetes Insipidus: A rare form of DI that occurs during pregnancy. It is caused by an enzyme produced by the placenta that breaks down ADH. This condition typically resolves after childbirth.

5. Dipsogenic Diabetes Insipidus: A type of DI associated with an abnormality in the thirst mechanism, located in the hypothalamus. It leads to excessive intake of fluids and subsequent suppression of ADH production.

6. Dehydration: A condition that occurs when the body loses more fluids than it takes in, leading to an insufficient amount of water to carry out normal bodily functions. Symptoms can include thirst, dark urine, fatigue, and dizziness.

7. Electrolyte: Minerals in the body, such as sodium, potassium, calcium, and magnesium, that are essential for regulating nerve and muscle function, hydrating the body, and balancing pH levels. Electrolyte imbalances can be a concern for individuals with DI.

8. Electrolyte Imbalance: A condition where the levels of electrolytes in the body are either too high or too low. This can result from excessive fluid loss due to DI and can lead to muscle weakness, irregular heartbeat, and other health issues.

9. Hyponatremia: A condition characterized by abnormally low sodium levels in the blood. This can occur if an individual with DI overhydrates without replenishing sodium, leading to water intoxication and potential neurological issues.

10. Nocturia: The need to wake up multiple times during the night to urinate. This is a common symptom of DI and can disrupt sleep quality and overall rest.

11. Polyuria: The production of abnormally large volumes of dilute urine. It is a primary symptom of DI, where individuals may produce 3 to 20 liters of urine per day.

12. Polydipsia: Excessive thirst and fluid intake. This is another hallmark symptom of DI, driven by the body's need to compensate for fluid lost through polyuria.

13. Desmopressin (DDAVP): A synthetic form of ADH that is used as a medication to treat central DI. It works by reducing the amount of urine produced by the kidneys and is available in various forms, such as tablets, nasal sprays, and injections.

14. Vasopressin: Another name for antidiuretic hormone (ADH). It plays a crucial role in the body's ability to regulate water balance and blood pressure.

15. Pituitary Gland: A small, pea-sized gland located at the base of the brain. It stores and releases ADH, among other hormones, and plays a vital role in regulating bodily functions.

16. Hypothalamus: A region of the brain that produces ADH and regulates various essential bodily functions, including temperature, thirst, and hunger. Damage or abnormalities in the hypothalamus can lead to DI.

17. Urinalysis: A laboratory test that analyzes urine samples to check for various substances and abnormalities. This test can help diagnose conditions like DI by measuring urine concentration and volume.

18. Serum Osmolality: A test that measures the concentration of particles in the blood. High serum osmolality can indicate dehydration, while low levels can suggest overhydration. This test helps monitor fluid balance and assess DI.

19. Water Deprivation Test: A diagnostic test used to determine the type of DI a person has. During the test, fluid intake is restricted to see how the body responds in terms of urine concentration and ADH release.

20. Hypernatremia: A condition in which sodium levels in the blood are higher than normal. This can occur when water loss exceeds sodium loss, often seen in cases of DI without adequate fluid intake.

21. Thirst Mechanism: A complex system regulated by the hypothalamus that triggers the sensation of thirst when the body needs more fluids. In dipsogenic DI, this mechanism can be faulty, leading to excessive fluid intake.

22. Hydration: The process of ensuring that the body has enough fluids to function properly. For individuals with DI, maintaining proper hydration is crucial to managing symptoms and preventing complications.

23. Hypokalemia: A condition characterized by low levels of potassium in the blood. It can lead to muscle weakness, cramping, and arrhythmias, and may be exacerbated by frequent urination in individuals with DI.

24. Chronic Fatigue: Persistent tiredness that is not relieved by rest and can impact daily functioning. Chronic fatigue may occur in individuals with DI due to nocturia and interrupted sleep patterns.

25. Cognitive Behavioral Therapy for Insomnia (CBT-I): A structured program that helps individuals address behaviors and thoughts that contribute to sleep problems. This therapy can be beneficial for those with DI experiencing insomnia due to nocturia.

26. Oral Rehydration Solution (ORS): A solution containing water, electrolytes, and sugar used to replenish fluids and minerals lost through excessive urination. ORS can be helpful for individuals with DI to maintain electrolyte balance.

27. Fluid Restriction: A controlled reduction in fluid intake, often used in medical settings to prevent overhydration. In DI, fluid restriction is managed carefully to avoid worsening dehydration or hyponatremia.

28. Medical Alert Bracelet: A wearable ID that provides essential information about an individual's medical condition. For individuals with DI, it can indicate their diagnosis and any emergency needs, such as the requirement for immediate access to water.

29. Hydration Apps: Mobile applications that help individuals track their water intake and set reminders to drink fluids throughout the day. These tools can be particularly useful for people with DI to maintain proper hydration.

30. 504 Plan: A formal plan developed in schools to ensure that a child with a medical condition receives the accommodations needed to participate fully in school activities. For children with DI, a 504 Plan may include allowances for frequent restroom breaks and water access.

31. Individualized Education Program (IEP): A plan designed to meet the educational needs of a child with a disability. For children with DI, an IEP may involve specific accommodations to manage symptoms and support learning.

32. Hypervolemia: An increase in blood volume due to excessive water intake without adequate sodium, which can lead to water retention and potential complications such as hyponatremia.

33. Rare Disease Advocacy: Efforts to raise awareness, improve research, and promote better policies for rare conditions, including DI.

These efforts can involve participation in support groups, sharing personal stories, and lobbying for legislative changes.

34. Restroom Access Accommodations: Adjustments made in schools or workplaces to allow individuals with DI to use the restroom as needed. These accommodations help prevent disruptions and promote comfort and productivity.

35. Telemedicine: The use of technology to provide healthcare services remotely. This can be especially helpful for individuals with DI to manage their condition through virtual consultations with healthcare providers.

36. Sleep Hygiene: Practices that contribute to better sleep quality, including maintaining a consistent sleep schedule, creating a comfortable sleep environment, and limiting stimulants before bedtime. These practices are essential for individuals with DI who struggle with nocturia.

37. Self-Advocacy: The practice of representing one's needs and interests, particularly in healthcare or educational settings. People with DI and their caregivers often need to advocate for appropriate treatment, accommodations, and support.

38. Fatigue Management: Strategies to mitigate the effects of tiredness, such as scheduling breaks, staying hydrated, and engaging in energy-boosting activities. This is particularly important for those with DI experiencing interrupted sleep due to nocturia.

39. Urine Concentration: The amount of solutes in the urine, which determines how concentrated or diluted it is. In DI, urine is often very diluted due to the body's inability to conserve water properly.

40. Hydration-Friendly Foods: Foods with high water content that contribute to overall hydration. Examples include cucumbers, watermelon, and lettuce, which can support fluid intake in addition to drinking water.

This glossary provides a comprehensive overview of the medical and condition-specific terms essential for understanding and managing Diabetes Insipidus. Familiarity with these terms will help individuals, caregivers, and healthcare professionals navigate DI management with greater confidence and clarity.

Appendix B: Resources

Navigating the complexities of Diabetes Insipidus (DI) can be challenging, but there are numerous resources available to provide support, information, and assistance. This appendix compiles websites, organizations, and support groups that can help individuals, caregivers, and families find reliable information, connect with others, and access medical and emotional support.

B.1 Educational Websites

These websites offer reliable and comprehensive information on DI, including its causes, symptoms, treatment options, and management tips.

1. National Institute of Diabetes and Digestive and Kidney Diseases (NIDDK)

- **Website**: www.niddk.nih.gov
- **Overview**: A government organization that provides authoritative resources on various health conditions, including DI. The site includes detailed articles, research findings, and patient education materials.
- **Best For**: General information, research updates, and educational resources.

2. Mayo Clinic

- **Website**: www.mayoclinic.org
- **Overview**: A reputable medical organization known for its in-depth medical articles. The Mayo Clinic website offers clear explanations of DI symptoms, causes, treatments, and prevention tips.
- **Best For**: Patient-friendly medical explanations and treatment overviews.

3. MedlinePlus

- **Website**: www.medlineplus.gov
- **Overview**: Managed by the National Library of Medicine, this resource offers information on various health conditions, including DI, with links to clinical trials, journal articles, and medical encyclopedias.
- **Best For**: Access to high-quality health information, clinical trial links, and related medical topics.

B.2 Organizations and Foundations

These organizations focus on supporting individuals with DI and other rare conditions. They provide advocacy, research funding, community building, and educational resources.

1. National Organization for Rare Disorders (NORD)

- **Website**: www.rarediseases.org
- **Overview**: NORD is dedicated to improving the lives of individuals with rare diseases. It offers information, advocacy tools, and support for those living with conditions like DI.
- **Best For**: Advocacy, rare disease information, and patient assistance programs.

2. The Pituitary Foundation

- **Website**: www.pituitary.org.uk
- **Overview**: This UK-based foundation focuses on pituitary gland disorders, including DI. The organization provides resources, patient stories, and support group information.
- **Best For**: Pituitary-related information, DI management, and support networks.

3. Hormone Health Network

- **Website**: www.hormone.org
- **Overview**: Provides educational resources on hormone-related conditions, including DI. The site features patient guides, FAQs, and hormone health tips.
- **Best For**: Hormone-related resources and understanding the endocrine system's impact on DI.

4. Diabetes Insipidus Foundation

- **Website**: www.diabetesinsipidus.org
- **Overview**: A dedicated organization focusing specifically on supporting individuals with DI. They offer educational materials, community forums, and fundraising for research.
- **Best For**: DI-focused resources, patient education, and research funding initiatives.

5. Endocrine Society

- **Website**: www.endocrine.org
- **Overview**: A global community of endocrinologists and healthcare providers dedicated to endocrine system research and education. The website includes patient resources and educational material on various conditions, including DI.
- **Best For**: Expert information on endocrine health and DI, educational webinars, and medical articles.

B.3 Support Groups and Forums

Connecting with others who share similar experiences can provide emotional support and practical advice. The following resources offer community support and forums for discussion.

1. Inspire

- **Website**: www.inspire.com
- **Overview**: An online health and wellness community with discussion boards dedicated to rare diseases and chronic health conditions. Users can share experiences, ask questions, and offer support to others with DI.
- **Best For**: Peer support, shared stories, and community interaction.

2. RareConnect

- **Website**: www.rareconnect.org
- **Overview**: A platform hosted by NORD and EURORDIS that connects people with rare diseases, including DI. Members can join forums, participate in discussions, and access multilingual resources.
- **Best For**: Global community engagement and connecting with other rare disease patients.

3. Facebook Support Groups

- **Platform**: Facebook
- **Overview**: Search for groups related to DI, such as "Diabetes Insipidus Support" or "Living with DI," to find online communities of individuals and families sharing experiences, advice, and support.

- **Best For**: Real-time interaction, advice sharing, and connecting with a broad range of DI patients and caregivers.

4. Reddit – r/rare_diseases

- **Website**: www.reddit.com/r/rare_diseases
- **Overview**: A subreddit dedicated to discussing rare diseases, including DI. Members share personal stories, ask questions, and offer support.
- **Best For**: Anonymity, sharing experiences, and learning from others facing similar challenges.

B.4 Resources for Children and Families

Managing DI in children can be particularly challenging. These resources cater specifically to families and young patients.

1. KidsHealth

- **Website**: www.kidshealth.org
- **Overview**: Provides child-friendly medical information and advice for parents. It offers articles on DI and how to support children with the condition.
- **Best For**: Parents seeking guidance on helping children manage DI.

2. Child Mind Institute

- **Website**: www.childmind.org
- **Overview**: While not DI-specific, this organization offers resources on how to support children dealing with medical conditions that can impact their mental health and social well-being.
- **Best For**: Parents and caregivers looking for strategies to support children's mental health.

3. Parent Support Groups

- **Local and Online Communities**: Check with local hospitals, community centers, or schools to find parent support groups that focus on rare conditions or general chronic illness management.
- **Best For**: Connecting with other parents and sharing practical advice for raising a child with DI.

B.5 Research and Advocacy

Advocacy and research play critical roles in raising awareness and promoting better treatment for DI. The following resources can help you stay informed and get involved.

1. ClinicalTrials.gov

- **Website**: www.clinicaltrials.gov
- **Overview**: A database of privately and publicly funded clinical studies conducted around the world. Search for ongoing and upcoming clinical trials related to DI to stay informed about potential new treatments and research developments.
- **Best For**: Information on clinical trials and research studies for DI.

2. Global Genes

- **Website**: www.globalgenes.org
- **Overview**: An organization dedicated to raising awareness and supporting rare disease communities. They provide toolkits, webinars, and educational resources to empower patients and advocates.
- **Best For**: Advocacy resources, educational materials, and networking opportunities.

3. EURORDIS – Rare Diseases Europe

- **Website**: www.eurordis.org
- **Overview**: A patient-driven alliance of organizations that represent rare disease patients in Europe. They offer resources, advocacy tools, and support for individuals with rare diseases, including DI.

- **Best For**: Advocacy and awareness efforts, particularly in Europe.

4. Genetic and Rare Diseases Information Center (GARD)

- **Website**: www.rarediseases.info.nih.gov
- **Overview**: A program of the National Center for Advancing Translational Sciences (NCATS) that provides information about rare and genetic diseases. GARD can offer detailed medical information on DI and other rare conditions.
- **Best For**: Comprehensive medical information and updates on rare diseases.

B.6 Emergency and Medical Support Resources

These resources are valuable for urgent medical needs and finding local medical assistance.

1. Medical Alert Services

- **Provider Examples**: MedicAlert Foundation (www.medicalert.org)
- **Overview**: Provides wearable medical alert bracelets or IDs that inform first responders of an individual's medical conditions, including DI. This service can be life-saving in emergencies.
- **Best For**: Emergency preparedness and immediate recognition of medical conditions.

2. Telehealth Services

- **Examples**: Teladoc (www.teladoc.com), Amwell (www.amwell.com)
- **Overview**: Telehealth platforms offer remote medical consultations for non-emergency medical needs. These services can be beneficial for managing DI symptoms and discussing treatment plans without leaving home.

- **Best For**: Access to healthcare professionals and continuity of care.

3. Local Emergency Services

- **Contact Information**: Save the phone numbers of local emergency rooms, urgent care centers, and pharmacies in your area. Having these contacts readily available can make a significant difference during an emergency related to DI.

This appendix provides a starting point for finding information, support, and community while managing Diabetes Insipidus. Whether you're seeking educational resources, community support, or ways to get involved in advocacy, these resources can guide and assist you throughout your journey.

Appendix C: Sample Hydration Log

Keeping a detailed hydration log is essential for individuals managing Diabetes Insipidus (DI) to monitor water intake, medication schedules, and symptoms. This appendix provides a comprehensive template that can be used to track these elements effectively. By maintaining a consistent log, you can identify patterns, ensure proper hydration, adhere to medication schedules, and share relevant data with healthcare providers for better management of DI.

C.1 Purpose of a Hydration Log

A hydration log helps individuals with DI to:

- **Track Daily Water Intake**: Monitor total fluid consumption throughout the day to ensure adequate hydration without over-hydration.
- **Document Medication Times**: Record the exact times medications are taken to maintain consistent treatment.
- **Identify Symptoms**: Keep a record of any symptoms experienced, such as excessive thirst, fatigue, or changes in urination, to help with symptom management and medical consultations.
- **Spot Patterns**: Analyze trends in hydration, medication effectiveness, and symptom triggers over time.

C.2 Template for Daily Hydration Log

Below is a template designed to help you track your hydration, medication, and symptoms throughout the day. Feel free to customize it to better suit your specific needs.

Sample Hydration Log Template

| Date: _____________ | Day of the Week: _____________ |

Time	Water Intake (mL)	Other Fluids (Type/ Amount)	Medication Taken (Type/ Dose)	Symptoms/ Notes	Urination Frequency
6:00 AM					
7:00 AM					
8:00 AM					
9:00 AM					
10:00 AM					
11:00 AM					
12:00 PM					
1:00 PM					

Time	Water Intake (mL)	Other Fluids (Type/ Amount)	Medication Taken (Type/ Dose)	Symptoms/ Notes	Urination Frequency
2:00 PM					
3:00 PM					
4:00 PM					
5:00 PM					
6:00 PM					
7:00 PM					
8:00 PM					
9:00 PM					
10:00 PM					

Daily Totals:

- **Total Water Intake (mL):** _____________
- **Total Other Fluids (mL):** _____________

- **Medications Taken**:
  - Name/Dose:

  ____

  - Time(s)   Taken:

  ____

Notes:

- Include any significant symptoms experienced, such as dizziness, extreme thirst, or fatigue.
- Note unusual changes in urination patterns (e.g., frequency, volume, color).

Overall Daily Observations:

- Did you feel adequately hydrated? (Yes/No) ____________
- Any significant changes compared to previous days? _____________________________________
- Energy levels: High/Medium/Low ___________

C.3 Guidelines for Using the Hydration Log

1. **Set a Schedule**: Decide on consistent times to log your water intake, medication, and symptoms throughout the day. Setting phone reminders can help maintain consistency.
2. **Be Accurate**: Measure fluid intake accurately using marked water bottles or measuring cups.
3. **Record Medications Promptly**: Write down the time medications are taken to monitor their effectiveness and consistency.
4. **Track Symptoms Honestly**: Document any symptoms as soon as they occur to provide a comprehensive record for review.

5. **Review Regularly**: At the end of each week, review the logs to identify any trends or areas for adjustment. Share these insights with your healthcare provider for tailored medical advice.

C.4 Sample Completed Log Entry
Date: 11/10/2024 | **Day of the Week**: Sunday

Time	Water Intake (mL)	Other Fluids (Type/Amount)	Medication Taken (Type/Dose)	Symptoms/Notes	Urination Frequency
6:00 AM	250			Woke up thirsty	1
7:00 AM	200		Desmopressin 0.1 mg		
8:00 AM	150			Feeling well	1
9:00 AM		150 (tea)		Slight fatigue	
10:00 AM	200				1
11:00 AM	100			Energy level stable	
12:00 PM	250				

Time	Water Intake (mL)	Other Fluids (Type/ Amount)	Medication Taken (Type/ Dose)	Symptoms/ Notes	Urination Frequency
1:00 PM	150			Minor thirst	1
2:00 PM	200				
3:00 PM		100 (juice)		No significant symptoms	1
4:00 PM	150				
5:00 PM	100			Started feeling slightly thirsty	2
6:00 PM	200				
7:00 PM	150				1
8:00 PM	150			Preparing for bed	

Time	Water Intake (mL)	Other Fluids (Type/ Amount)	Medication Taken (Type/ Dose)	Symptoms/ Notes	Urination Frequency
9:00 PM	100			Reduced intake for sleep prep	
10:00 PM				Asleep by 10:30 PM	

Daily Totals:

- **Total Water Intake (mL):** 1950 mL
- **Total Other Fluids (mL):** 250 mL
- **Medications Taken:**
    - Desmopressin 0.1 mg at 7:00 AM

Overall Daily Observations:

- Did you feel adequately hydrated? Yes
- Any significant changes compared to previous days? Maintained hydration well; slight afternoon fatigue.
- Energy levels: Medium

Note: Modify the hydration log template based on your needs, such as adding sections for food intake, physical activity, or sleep quality for a more holistic overview of how DI management affects your daily life.

This detailed tracking will provide valuable insights for both self-management and medical consultations.

Appendix D: Frequently Asked Questions

Understanding and managing Diabetes Insipidus (DI) can come with many questions, whether you are newly diagnosed, caring for someone with the condition, or looking to optimize your lifestyle. This appendix addresses common questions regarding DI, its treatment, and lifestyle adjustments to provide clarity and guidance.

D.1 General Questions About Diabetes Insipidus

Q1: What is the difference between Diabetes Insipidus and diabetes mellitus?

- **Answer**: Although both conditions share the word "diabetes," they are fundamentally different. **Diabetes Insipidus (DI)** is a disorder related to water balance in the body, characterized by excessive urination and thirst due to inadequate ADH production or kidney response. **Diabetes mellitus**, on the other hand, is a metabolic condition related to high blood sugar levels caused by insulin deficiency or resistance. The two conditions affect the body in different ways and have distinct causes and treatments.

Q2: What causes Diabetes Insipidus?

- **Answer**: DI can be caused by different factors:
    - **Central Diabetes Insipidus (CDI)**: Results from damage to the hypothalamus or pituitary gland, which affects ADH production or release. Causes include head injuries, surgery, tumors, or genetic disorders.
    - **Nephrogenic Diabetes Insipidus (NDI)**: Occurs when the kidneys do not respond properly to ADH. This can be due to genetic factors, chronic kidney disease, or certain medications such as lithium.

- ◦ **Gestational Diabetes Insipidus**: Occurs during pregnancy due to an enzyme from the placenta breaking down ADH.
- ◦ **Dipsogenic Diabetes Insipidus**: Results from an abnormal thirst mechanism in the hypothalamus that leads to excessive fluid intake and suppressed ADH production.

Q3: Is DI a rare condition?

- **Answer**: Yes, DI is considered a rare condition compared to diabetes mellitus. Central and nephrogenic DI are the most common types, while gestational and dipsogenic DI are rarer.

Q4: Can DI be cured?

- **Answer**: While DI cannot be "cured" in most cases, it can often be managed effectively with proper treatment and lifestyle adjustments. The prognosis depends on the underlying cause. For example, DI resulting from a temporary condition, such as gestational DI or a post-surgical issue, may resolve on its own.

D.2 Questions About Treatment and Medications

Q5: What is the main treatment for Central Diabetes Insipidus?

- **Answer**: The primary treatment for **Central DI** is **desmopressin (DDAVP)**, a synthetic form of ADH that helps reduce urine production and control excessive thirst. Desmopressin can be administered as a tablet, nasal spray, or injection.

Q6: Are there different treatment options for Nephrogenic Diabetes Insipidus?

- **Answer**: Yes, treatment for **Nephrogenic DI** typically involves:
    - **Low-sodium diet**: Reducing salt intake helps minimize urine production.
    - **Diuretics**: Surprisingly, certain diuretics, such as thiazide diuretics, can help decrease urine output in NDI by altering kidney function.
    - **Adequate hydration**: Ensuring regular water intake is essential.
    - **NSAIDs (e.g., indomethacin)**: Sometimes used to reduce urine output by inhibiting prostaglandin production.

Q7: How is Gestational DI managed?

- **Answer**: **Gestational DI** is managed similarly to central DI, often with **desmopressin**, as the underlying issue is the breakdown of ADH during pregnancy. The condition usually resolves after childbirth.

Q8: Can I take desmopressin every day?

- **Answer**: Yes, **desmopressin** can be taken daily as prescribed by a healthcare provider. The dosage and frequency will vary based on individual needs and response to the medication. It is essential to follow medical advice closely to avoid potential side effects, such as water retention and low sodium levels (hyponatremia).

Q9: What are the potential side effects of desmopressin?

- **Answer**: Common side effects of **desmopressin** include headaches, nausea, mild flushing, and abdominal cramps. A serious but rare side effect is **hyponatremia** (low sodium levels), which can cause confusion, seizures, or coma if not managed. Monitoring fluid intake and symptoms is crucial.

D.3 Questions About Lifestyle and Daily Management
Q10: How much water should someone with DI drink daily?

- **Answer**: The amount of water needed varies depending on the severity of DI and other individual factors. Generally, people with DI need to drink enough water to match their fluid loss and prevent dehydration. This could mean drinking several liters a day. It is essential to follow a personalized hydration plan advised by a healthcare provider.

Q11: Can people with DI exercise safely?

- **Answer**: Yes, individuals with DI can exercise safely with proper precautions:
    - **Hydrate before, during, and after exercise** to prevent dehydration.
    - **Choose moderate-intensity activities** and avoid exercising in extreme heat to minimize excessive sweating.
    - **Listen to your body** and stop if you feel lightheaded or overly fatigued.

Q12: How does DI affect sleep, and what can be done to improve sleep quality?

- **Answer**: **Nocturia** (frequent nighttime urination) is a common issue in DI, which can disrupt sleep. To improve sleep quality:
  - **Limit fluid intake** a couple of hours before bedtime.
  - **Ensure medications** are taken at a time that aligns with sleep needs.
  - **Create a sleep-friendly environment** with low light and minimal noise to help with falling back asleep after waking.

Q13: Are there specific foods that can help manage DI symptoms?

- **Answer**: While no foods can cure DI, certain dietary choices can help manage symptoms:
  - **Water-rich foods**: Include cucumbers, watermelon, and oranges to aid hydration.
  - **Low-sodium meals**: Limit foods high in sodium to avoid increased thirst and excessive urine production.
  - **Balanced nutrition**: Maintain a diet rich in essential vitamins and minerals to support overall health and energy levels.

Q14: Can children with DI participate in normal activities?

- **Answer**: Yes, with proper management, children with DI can participate in regular activities. Ensure they:
  - **Stay hydrated** throughout the day, especially during physical activities.
  - **Have easy access to water and restrooms** at school or during extracurricular activities.

- ○ **Communicate their needs** with teachers, coaches, and caregivers to receive appropriate accommodations.

Q15: What accommodations can be made at school or work for someone with DI?

- **Answer**: Accommodations for individuals with DI may include:
    - ○ **Unlimited restroom access** to prevent disruptions and maintain comfort.
    - ○ **Permission to carry a water bottle** for continuous hydration.
    - ○ **Flexible scheduling** to manage symptoms, especially if they impact energy levels or focus.

D.4 Questions About Long-Term Management and Support
Q16: How often should I see a doctor for DI management?

- **Answer**: Regular follow-ups are essential for effective DI management. It is recommended to visit your healthcare provider every 6 to 12 months or as advised to monitor symptoms, treatment effectiveness, and potential complications.

Q17: Can DI lead to other health complications?

- **Answer**: If DI is not managed properly, it can lead to **dehydration** and **electrolyte imbalances**, which can have severe consequences. Chronic dehydration can affect kidney function and overall well-being. Maintaining proper hydration and regular medical check-ups helps mitigate these risks.

Q18: What should I do if I experience a sudden increase in symptoms?

- **Answer**: If you experience a sudden or unexplained increase in symptoms, such as excessive thirst and urination or signs of dehydration despite treatment, contact your healthcare provider immediately. Adjustments to medication or additional tests may be necessary to identify the cause.

Q19: Are there any support groups for people with DI?

- **Answer**: Yes, there are support groups available both online and locally where individuals with DI can connect and share their experiences. Websites like **Inspire**, **RareConnect**, and DI-specific groups on social media platforms provide valuable peer support and resources.

Q20: How can I educate my friends and family about my condition?

- **Answer**: To help friends and family understand DI:
  - **Provide clear, simple explanations** of what DI is and how it affects you.
  - **Share educational resources** from trusted medical websites or brochures provided by healthcare providers.
  - **Discuss practical ways they can help**, such as recognizing signs of dehydration or supporting your hydration and medication routines.

This appendix aims to address common questions related to DI, ensuring that individuals and caregivers have the information they need to manage the condition confidently and effectively. For further guidance, always consult with healthcare professionals familiar with your unique needs.

<u>Message from the Author:</u>

I hope you enjoyed this book, I love astrology and knew there was not a book such as this out on the shelf. I love metaphysical items as well. Please check out my other books:

-Life of Government Benefits

-My life of Hell

-My life with Hydrocephalus

-Red Sky

-World Domination:Woman's rule

-World Domination:Woman's Rule 2: The War

-Life and Banishment of Apophis: book 1

-The Kidney Friendly Diet

-The Ultimate Hemp Cookbook

-Creating a Dispensary(legally)

-Cleanliness throughout life: the importance of showering from childhood to adulthood.

-Strong Roots: The Risks of Overcoddling children

-Hemp Horoscopes: Cosmic Insights and Earthly Healing

- Celestial Hemp Navigating the Zodiac: Through the Green Cosmos

-Astrological Hemp: Aligning The Stars with Earth's Ancient Herb

-The Astrological Guide to Hemp: Stars, Signs, and Sacred Leaves

-Green Growth: Innovative Marketing Strategies for your Hemp Products and Dispensary

-Cosmic Cannabis

-Astrological Munchies

-Henry The Hemp

-Zodiacal Roots: The Astrological Soul Of Hemp

- **Green Constellations: Intersection of Hemp and Zodiac**

-Hemp in The Houses: An astrological Adventure Through The Cannabis Galaxy

-Galactic Ganja Guide

Heavenly Hemp

Zodiac Leaves

Doctor Who Astrology

Cannastrology

Stellar Satvias and Cosmic Indicas

Celestial Cannabis: A Zodiac Journey

AstroHerbology: The Sky and The Soil: Volume 1

AstroHerbology:Celestial Cannabis:Volume 2

Cosmic Cannabis Cultivation

The Starry Guide to Herbal Harmony: Volume 1

The Starry Guide to Herbal Harmony: Cannabis Universe: Volume 2

Yugioh Astrology: Astrological Guide to Deck, Duels and more

Nightmare Mansion: Echoes of The Abyss

Nightmare Mansion 2: Legacy of Shadows

Nightmare Mansion 3: Shadows of the Forgotten

Nightmare Mansion 4: Echoes of the Damned

The Life and Banishment of Apophis: Book 2

Nightmare Mansion: Halls of Despair

Healing with Herb: Cannabis and Hydrocephalus

Planetary Pot: Aligning with Astrological Herbs: Volume 1

Fast Track to Freedom: 30 Days to Financial Independence Using AI, Assets, and Agile Hustles

Cosmic Hemp Pathways

How to Become Financially Free in 30 Days: 10,000 Paths to Prosperity

Zodiacal Herbage: Astrological Insights: Volume 1

Nightmare Mansion: Whispers in the Walls

The Daleks Invade Atlantis

Henry the hemp and Hydrocephalus

10X The Kidney Friendly Diet
Cannabis Universe: Adult coloring book
Hemp Astrology: The Healing Power of the Stars
Zodiacal Herbage: Astrological Insights: Cannabis Universe: Volume 2
<u>**Planetary Pot: Aligning with Astrological Herbs: Cannabis Universes: Volume 2**</u>
Doctor Who Meets the Replicators and SG-1: The Ultimate Battle for Survival
Nightmare Mansion: Curse of the Blood Moon
<u>**The Celestial Stoner: A Guide to the Zodiac**</u>
Cosmic Pleasures: Sex Toy Astrology for Every Sign
Hydrocephalus Astrology: Navigating the Stars and Healing Waters
Lapis and the Mischievous Chocolate Bar

Celestial Positions: Sexual Astrology for Every Sign
Apophis's Shadow Work Journal: : A Journey of Self-Discovery and Healing
Kinky Cosmos: Sexual Kink Astrology for Every Sign
Digital Cosmos: The Astrological Digimon Compendium
Stellar Seeds: The Cosmic Guide to Growing with Astrology
Apophis's Daily Gratitude Journal

Cat Astrology: Feline Mysteries of the Cosmos
The Cosmic Kama Sutra: An Astrological Guide to Sexual Positions
Unleash Your Potential: A Guided Journal Powered by AI Insights
Whispers of the Enchanted Grove

Cosmic Pleasures: An Astrological Guide to Sexual Kinks
369, 12 Manifestation Journal

Whisper of the nocturne journal(blank journal for writing or drawing)

The Boogey Book

Locked In Reflection: A Chastity Journey Through Locktober

Generating Wealth Quickly:

How to Generate $100,000 in 24 Hours

Star Magic: Harness the Power of the Universe

The Flatulence Chronicles: A Fart Journal for Self-Discovery

The Doctor and The Death Moth

Seize the Day: A Personal Seizure Tracking Journal

The Ultimate Boogeyman Safari: A Journey into the Boogie World and Beyond

Whispers of Samhain: 1,000 Spells of Love, Luck, and Lunar Magic: Samhain Spell Book

Apophis's guides:

Witch's Spellbook Crafting Guide for Halloween

<u>Frost & Flame: The Enchanted Yule Grimoire of 1000 Winter Spells</u>

<u>The Ultimate Boogey Goo Guide & Spooky Activities for Halloween Fun</u>

Harmony of the Scales: A Libra's Spellcraft for Balance and Beauty

The Enchanted Advent: 36 Days of Christmas Wonders

Nightmare Mansion: The Labyrinth of Screams

Harvest of Enchantment: 1,000 Spells of Gratitude, Love, and Fortune for Thanksgiving

The Boogey Chronicles: A Journal of Nightly Encounters and Shadowy Secrets

The 12 Days of Financial Freedom: A Step-by-Step Christmas Countdown to Transform Your Finances

Sigil of the Eternal Spiral Blank Journal

A Christmas Feast: Timeless Recipes for Every Meal

Holiday Stress-Free Solutions: A Survival Guide to Thriving During the Festive Season

Yu-Gi-Oh! Holiday Gifting Mastery: The Ultimate Guide for Fans and Newcomers Alike

Holiday Harmony: A Hydrocephalus Survival Guide for the Festive Season

Celestial Craft: The Witch's Almanac for 2025 – A Cosmic Guide to Manifestations, Moons, and Mystical Events

Doctor Who: The Toymaker's Winter Wonderland

Tulsa King Unveiled: A Thrilling Guide to Stallone's Mafia Masterpiece

Pendulum Craft: A Complete Guide to Crafting and Using Personalized Divination Tools

Nightmare Mansion: Santa's Eternal Eve

Starlight Noel: A Cosmic Journey through Christmas Mysteries

The Dark Architect: Unlocking the Blueprint of Existence

Surviving the Embrace: The Ultimate Guide to Encounters with The Hugging Molly

The Enchanted Codex: Secrets of the Craft for Witches, Wiccans, and Pagans

Harvest of Gratitude: A Complete Thanksgiving Guide

Yuletide Essentials: A Complete Guide to an Authentic and Magical Christmas

Celestial Smokes: A Cosmic Guide to Cigars and Astrology

If you want solar for your home go here: https://www.harborso-lar.live/apophisenterprises/

Get Some Tarot cards: https://www.makeplayingcards.com/sell/
apophis-occult-shop

<u>**Get some shirts: https://www.bonfire.com/store/apophis-shirt-emporium/**</u>

<u>Instagrams:</u>
@apophis_enterprises,
@apophisbookemporium,
@apophisscardshop
Twitter: @apophisenterpr1
 Tiktok:@apophisenterprise
Youtube: @sg1fan23477, @FiresideRetreatKingdom
Hive: @sg1fan23477
CheeLee: @SG1fan23477

Podcast: Apophis Chat Zone: https://open.spotify.com/show/5zXbrCLEV2xzCp8ybrfHsk?si=fb4d4fdbdce44dec

Newsletter: https://apophiss-newsletter-27c897.beehiiv.com/